Critical praise for
The What's Happening to My Body? Book for Boys:

"Madaras's down-to-earth, conversational treatment of a topic that remains taboo in many families provides answers to all the basic questions about the physical and emotional changes of male puberty."
                                                    —*The Washington Post*

"Madaras demonstrates great sensitivity to the turbulent feelings and embarrassments inherent in the subject [of puberty]....Her facility for presenting information in a non-patronizing, well-organized manner is evident."
                                        —American Library Association

"Madaras seems to have an important gift as a sex educator that comes through clearly in her writing....She does with her book what all educators should strive to do—get students to think."
                                                        —*Siecus Report*

"You get a sense that [Madaras] understands the turmoil of the young teenager who is grasping for answers....This book is must reading."
                                        —Ralph I. Lopez, M.D.
                                        Associate Professor of Pediatrics
                                        Cornell Medical School

"One of the most complete, well-written, and clearly illustrated sex and health education texts to come off the press."
                                                    —*Arkansas Democrat*

OTHER BOOKS BY LYNDA MADARAS

My Body, My Self: The "What's Happening to My Body?" Workbook for Girls with Area Madaras

My Feelings, My Self: Lynda Madaras' Growing-Up Guide for Girls with Area Madaras

The "What's Happening to My Body?" Book for Girls with Area Madaras

Lynda Madaras Talks to Teens About AIDS: An Essential Guide for Parents, Teachers and Young People

Womancare: A Gynecological Guide to Your Body with Jane Patterson, M.D.

Woman Doctor: The Education of Jane Patterson, M.D. with Jane Patterson, M.D.

Great Expectations with Leigh Adams

The Alphabet Connection with Pam Palewicz-Rousseau

Child's Play

THE WHAT'S HAPPENING TO MY BODY?
BOOK FOR BOYS
NEW EDITION

*A Growing Up Guide
for Parents and Sons*

LYNDA MADARAS
with DANE SAAVEDRA

Drawings by Jackie Aher

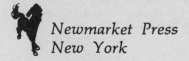

Newmarket Press
New York

OPM   30   29   28   27   26   25

Library of Congress Cataloging-in-Publication Data

Madaras, Lynda.
  The what's happening to my body? book for boys.

  Bibliography: p.
  Includes index.
  Summary: Discusses the changes that take place in a boy's body during puberty, including information on the body's changing size and shape, the growth spurt, reproductive organs, pubic hair, beards, pimples, voice changes, wet dreams, and puberty in girls.
  1. Adolescent boys—Growth. 2. Adolescent boys—Physiology. 3. Puberty. 4. Sex instruction for boys. [1. Sex instruction for boys. 2. Puberty. 3. Adolescent boys] I. Saavedra, Dane. II. Aher, Jackie, ill.
III. Title.
RJ143.M33 1987   613.9'53   87-28116
ISBN 1-55704-002-8
ISBN 0-937858-99-4 (pbk.)

Quantity Purchases
Companies, professional groups, clubs and other organizations may qualify for special terms when ordering quantities of this title. For information contact: Special Sales Dept., Newmarket Press, 18 East 48th Street, New York, New York 10017, or call (212) 832-3575.

Manufactured in the United States of America

New Edition

CONTENTS

LIST OF ILLUSTRATIONS

Foreword to the New Edition

by Ralph I. Lopez, M.D.

For nearly 20 years, my practice has been devoted solely to the care of teenagers. I begin to see boys and girls when they reach 12 years of age, and provide them with care through their college years. Several years ago, I had the opportunity to review Lynda Madaras's *What's Happening To My Body? Book for Girls.* I found it an ideal book for answering the questions of girls entering puberty — answering these questions, moreover, in a way that enabled parents and daughters to converse with one another about sexual topics.

Yet it was evident that another book was needed — one to similarly give young boys the facts. This void was filled by the arrival of Ms. Madaras's own *The What's Happening To My Body? Book for Boys.* With it, Ms. Madaras fulfilled the implicit promise of her preceding volume. In my foreword to its first edition, I called the *Boys* book "must reading."

"She doesn't mince her words," I wrote, "and you get a sense that she understands the turmoil of the young teenager who is grasping for answers." Now I have been given the opportunity to make a few comments about this new edition.

One might think that there would be little new to say in the way of sexual information. But the chapters appended here — on sexual intercourse and childbirth, on sexually transmitted diseases, and on romantic and sexual feelings — are a welcome addition. As in the first edition, the reader is introduced to these subjects with a combination of honesty and straight talk that is the only way to reach the questioning adolescent mind.

Both the parents and teenagers of this generation seem to operate on the fantastic assumption that kids today somehow "know it all" when it comes to sex. The topic is certainly bandied about so casually, even frivolously, by the mass media that one might think it were so. Yet, as a doctor providing medical care to both boys and girls — of all races and religions, of every conceivable economic bracket, and all living in a major urban center—I am constantly amazed at the discrepancy between street fiction and fact, between word-of-mouth myth and reality, where sexual topics are concerned. It is certainly true that teenagers have much more information available to them. But we lose sight of the fact that is the nature of teenagers to brag about what they *think* they know, and to maintain a reluctant silence when offered the opportunity to ask those "embarrassing questions." In this book Lynda Madaras answers "the embarrassing questions" with direct and specific language—unembarrassedly.

I strongly urge parents to read Ms. Madaras's book to get a sense of the questions that teenage boys will ask—or at least *want* to ask. Though most parents are full of good intentions, they often shy away from that famous "heart-to-heart talk" with their children. And yet the question that most boys are forever asking me is simply "Am I normal?," "Is this normal?," "What's normal?," or words to that effect. They ask me about their height, their rate of growth, their voice-changes, and — if they dare—their genitals. I try to give them reassurance that their problems are, indeed, normal.

Ms. Madaras's book not only handles these questions, but an additional concern as well. In today's sexual climate, the worries of teenagers (and adults, too) about "the sexual jungle out there" are quite legitimate. "Do you get this disease if you do this?," I am asked. "Is it safe to...?" The anxieties of adolescence and emerging sexuality are difficult enough without the added fears of disease and death. This new edition handles these and other fears so well that I suspect many parents will find themselves peeking at the book for answers to their own unvoiced questions. They may wish to get their own copies for that reason, as well as to prepare for their son's questions. Otherwise they may be forced to wait until their son has finished with his copy, which is likely to be dog-eared with use.

Ralph I. Lopez, M.D.
Clinical Associate Professor of Pediatrics
and Attending Physician: Adolescent Clinic,
The New York Hospital – Cornell Medical School

INTRODUCTION FOR PARENTS: Why I Wrote This Book

Toward the end of the school year, I give each of the boys and girls in my sex-education classes a raw egg and a homework assignment that goes something like this.

We're going to play a game. For one week, this egg is your baby. Fortunately for you, you don't have to feed it or change its diapers or get a job in order to earn enough money to buy clothes for it and put a roof over its head. But other than this, you have to take care of the egg as if it really were a baby and you were responsible for it. This means that you can't leave it alone unless you arrange for someone else to watch it while you're gone.

I'm giving you a break, though. I'm going to say that your babies are old enough to sleep through the night. This means that your baby won't wake up at two or three in the morning, howling to be fed—an unfortunate habit that most real babies have during the first months of their lives.

As I say, your babies are old enough to sleep through the night, so all you have to do at bedtime is give baby a kiss and tuck him or her (you decide which it is) into the refrigerator. You don't have to worry about baby again until the next morning. But in the morning, you have to remember to take your baby out of the fridge and bring it to school.

When you forget to bring your lunch money or gym clothes or math book to school, nothing *too* terrible happens. But if you forget to bring your baby to school even once, it's dead and you're out of the game. Not only that, but if any member of the Child Welfare League finds a neglected baby—that is, a baby left unattended—that baby will be confiscated.

I am president of the Child Welfare League, and all the staff and teachers are members. So is every student in the school, which means that you, too, are a member of the League. You are sworn to protect the welfare of all egg babies, and as your president, I expect every member of the League to be extremely vigilant about confiscating unattended and neglected babies.

At the end of the week, I will take all surviving babies and their parents out to lunch.

Good luck!

P.S. The parents of confiscated babies will *not* be taken to lunch.

The egg babies in my classes do not fare well. Most die of multiple fractures soon after birth. Some rot. Others simply disappear in the eternity of time that is a child's week. Still others are confiscated by the (at times) alarmingly zealous junior members of the Child Welfare League.

One year there was even a baby who committed suicide—at least that's how the baby's "father" attempted to explain the demise of his egg. It seems this baby had, "all by itself," totally of its own accord, rolled off his desk in the middle of French class. The father tried to argue that the parent of a suicidal baby deserved to be taken out to lunch. Being a hard-hearted lot, the class refused to acknowledge his point.

So far, in six years of teaching these classes, I have only had to take two kids and their egg babies out to lunch (and there was some talk in one case about a fresh egg having been substituted for a broken baby).

I must admit that I get a real kick out of watching what goes on at school in the week during this homework assignment. There are always a couple of boys who try to get one of the girls to care for their babies because "taking care of babies is woman's work." It warms the cockles of my heart to see this tactic fall flat on its face. But there are also the boys who take their parenting very seriously. I'll see them out on the patio at lunch, four or five boys eating together, with their egg babies resting on a strip of soft velvet in the center of the table. They'll be chatting away about the various bumps and cracks their babies have just narrowly escaped, sounding for all the world like the congregations of young mothers who gather over baby strollers in the park to compare notes and trade tales of barely averted childhood disasters.

Within a day or so after I have given the assignment, the egg babies have taken on definite personalities. Carefully crayoned features appear on their formerly blank faces, and the "parents" have all named their babies. Ingenious cribs and cradles and carriages have been fashioned. Once, a boy brought his egg to school in one of those plastic, oval-shaped containers that some panty hose comes in—a "self-contained life-support capsule," the proud father explained. It always surprises me that it is not just the younger kids but also the older teens—and the boys as well as the girls—who get involved in the game and set about designing these cribs and cradles and such for their babies. The sight of a hulking fifteen-year-old with the build of a football player trotting across the campus with his egg baby tenderly tucked in a carefully constructed milk carton cradle never fails to amaze me.

This homework assignment comes at the end of a section of the curriculum in which the kids, at least the ones in my older classes, tackle such thorny issues as:

- How old should you be before you have sex?
- How do you know if you're ready for sex?
- Should you wait until you're married?
- How to say no to sex
- Birth control
- The fact that birth control isn't 100 percent effective

- Abortion
- Parenthood
- Sexuality and the responsibility for the lives and feelings of others

The thinking behind the egg baby assignment is, of course, to give kids some idea of the realities of and the responsibilities involved in parenthood. I suppose that at the heart of it, this assignment is really nothing more than an old-fashioned moral object lesson, something along the lines of the stories my grandmother would tell in which children, though warned not to, would skate on thin-ice ponds and drown. Although I heard these tales often, I did venture out on a few thin-ice ponds in my time, and, all in all, the warnings did not have a profound effect on me. So I am not naive enough to think that giving kids raw eggs to take care of for a week is going to make them stop in the middle of the throes of teenage passion and think about forgoing sex altogether or at least using birth control. Still, I figure it can't hurt. We do, after all, have a virtual epidemic of teenage pregnancies in this country, over a million babies born to teenage mothers each year. One-half of today's teenagers, some 11 million kids, are sexually active. Four out of every ten of today's fourteen-year-old girls will become pregnant at least once during their teenage years. Given these facts, anything—even a long shot like the egg baby assignment—seems worth a try.

Even if this assignment never prevents a single teenage pregnancy, the kids have fun and I like to think they learn something from it. But more important, perhaps, is that each year I learn, or relearn, something about the confusing contradictions young boys must deal with as they move into manhood.

The boys who are out on the patio clucking over their babies, the football players who have spent hours lovingly fashioning their cribs and cradles, are the very same boys who come up to me before class, giggling and pushing at me dog-eared copies of whatever racy, adolescent paperback novel has been making the rounds of late. "Read this, read this," they insist, the books open to pages on which "the good parts" have been underlined in red.

During the past couple of years, it's been Nick Carter novels. Possibly you aren't familiar with these, and I must admit that I have never read much more than "the good parts" of any Nick Carter novel. Apparently, though, Nick is some sort of detective or international spy or CIA operative. Nick and his fellow heroes of this particular literary genre are quite a bunch of guys. They have all sorts of thrilling adventures and narrow escapes. They are, each and every one, precision marksmen. They generally drive very fast, very expensive, very red sports cars. They are well-versed in obscure martial arts, which they regularly apply to various thugs and scoundrels of a vaguely Mafioso, Communist ilk. And of course truth, justice, the American way, and our heroes always triumph in the end. But all the intrigue and rather convoluted plots are just so much window dressing, merely something to hang "the good parts" on—for what the Nick Carter novels and the others of the genre are really about is *sex*.

Curiously enough, Nick and his literary counterparts, at least in my spotty readings, rarely seem to make the first sexual moves. Instead, it's the women who "come on" to them (a rather effective device for sidestepping the old fear-of-rejection problem).

There is nothing in the least bit shy or retiring about the ladies Nick encounters. They are a most lascivious lot. The women in these novels are forever ripping open their blouses and begging our hero to have his way with them. The hero, being a gentleman, obliges. There is a curiously Victorian coyness to the lurid detailing of these sexual exploits. It's always the hero's "manhood," his "organ," his "hardness," or his throbbing pulsating "member" that so delights the ladies and their "wet openness"—never anything so clinical, explicit, or mundane as a "penis" or a "vagina."

These sexual gymnastics often continue for several pages. As I said, Nick and his cohorts are quite a bunch of guys. Often the episodes wind to a close with the ladies expressing gratitude for the wonderful satisfaction our hero has provided and declaring their undying love for him, although as far as I've been able to determine the women and the hero rarely, if ever, meet up again.

I am not normally one to rain on anybody's parade, but when the boys in my classes ask me to read the underlined sections of books like these, I figure that they're asking for some sort of reaction, that they want to know what I think. So I tell them. I do my best to avoid being sarcastic—that clearly isn't the tack called for here. I explain that neither my sex life nor the sex life of anyone else I know on the planet proceeds along the lines described in these books. We discuss what's unreal about the sexual encounters in Nick's life and why the author chose to portray them in this light. We talk about the real-life fears and uncertainties most people have in regard to sex, about sexuality and the emotional feelings involved in being sexual with another person. From an educational point of view, we get a lot of mileage out of old Nick.

The issue I'm trying to get at here is that this culture poses some rather tricky problems for young boys trying to find their way into manhood. On the one hand, they have a tender, caring side—the side I see so clearly when they're essentially "playing dolls" with egg babies. On the other hand, they are confronted with all these thrilling and titillating images of a conquering, tough-guy male sexuality, which doesn't seem to allow much room for anybody's being at all tender or caring. It must be rather difficult to reconcile making a cradle for your egg baby with the sagas of Nick Carter. It must be very hard for a boy to sort all this out, and this undoubtedly accounts for a large portion of the adolescent male angst. Of course, what I'm talking about here isn't any great revelation. We all know that during childhood boys generally are allowed some room, given some social permission, to demonstrate or act out their tender side. And we all know that at adolescence they begin to move into the strange world of male adulthood in which, if Nick is to be believed, "real men" are not noted for their tenderness, "real men" don't cry or ever feel uncertain about who they are or what they're supposed to do, "real men" always know the right sexual moves to make, "real men" are always knowledgeable and supremely confident about sex and life in general.

To top it all off, just as they're moving from childhood into this confusing world of manhood, all these strange changes start happening to their bodies. And chances are that nobody around them seems willing to explain these changes in any but the most cursory way, if at all. In fact, the message that boys are getting is that somehow they're supposed to *know* about these things, for one of the main tenets of the male mystique is that guys, or at least "real men," automatically know everything about anything that has to do with sex.

In recent years, there's been a great deal of heated public

debate about the nature of sex education in our nation's schools, much of it generated by conservative parents who feel that sex education belongs in the home, and that the sexual morality implied in these classes is not up to snuff. More liberal parents have taken up the banner in response to these attacks and have loudly and ferociously defended sex-education programs. You may be a conservative or you may be a liberal. You may be on one side or the other of this debate. Being a sex-education teacher, I have my own, rather predictable, point of view on the issue. But I'm willing to concede that there are valid points to be made on each side.

In general, I think that public debate on an issue like this is a good thing. I do worry, though, that it leaves parents with the impression that there is, in fact, something to debate about, that there *are* sex-education programs throughout our nation's schools. Unfortunately, this is not the case. According to one recent survey, fewer than 15 percent of the teenagers in this country are exposed to a comprehensive sex-education program. If you've been assuming, as many parents do—especially in the wake of all this debate—that at school your boy is getting the information he needs about the sexual changes of puberty, chances are you're wrong. In most schools, sex education still consists of the kind of thing that happened when we were kids. One day, usually in the sixth grade, all the boys are mysteriously sent out to the playground for an extra "free" period, to play baseball or whatever sport is in season. The girls are herded into the auditorium and shown a film, generally produced by one of the sanitary napkin and tampon manufacturers, in which butterflies flitter through uteri and in which menstruation and the need to use these various menstrual products are explained.

The schools simply aren't doing the job we parents, for better or worse, imagine that they're doing. For the average boy, home isn't much of a source of information either. Most of the girls in my classes have been the recipients of at least one rather nervous and embarrassed "talk" from their parents (as a rule, their mothers) about menstruation, the hallmark of female puberty. But there are very few boys in my classes whose parents (either the mother or the father) have talked with them about ejaculation, the hallmark of male puberty, or about spontaneous erections, masturbation, wet dreams, or any of the other physical realities of male puberty. I'm not sure why we have decided that it's important to talk to our daughters about puberty but not so important to talk to our sons. Perhaps it has something to do with the fact that our daughter's first menstruation requires at least some sort of minimal parental response—someone's got to buy her a box of sanitary napkins or tampons and tell her how they're used and not to flush them down the toilet. When a boy ejaculates for the first time, we don't have to rush out to the store for anything, and we don't have to worry about him clogging up the plumbing. It's a lot easier to ignore our sons' "coming of age" than it is to ignore our daughters'.

Or perhaps it has to do with the fact that once our daughters begin to menstruate regularly, they become, for the first time, capable of getting pregnant. This fact alone seems to convince many parents that their daughters deserve some sex education. And yet, girls don't get pregnant by themselves. As my mother used to say, "It takes two to tango," although she was never talking about dancing when she said this.

Or maybe it's just the old male mystique, the belief that boys automatically know everything they need to know about sex. Few parents would actually argue that boys will magically understand what's happening to their bodies without someone telling them. But many parents have the attitude that puberty isn't really a "big deal" for boys. There's a popular idea in our culture that it's only girls who are embarrassed, anxious, and worried about the physical changes of puberty.

You couldn't prove it by me. In my sex-education classes, we play a game called Everything You Ever Wanted to Know About Sex and Puberty but Were Too Embarrassed to Ask, which involves a locked question box to which kids can anonymously submit questions. At the end of each class, I open the box, read out loud the questions that have accumulated that week, and answer them as best I can. The questions come printed in block letters (to disguise the handwriting), and the paper on which they're written has inevitably been folded about ten times into a tiny little packet. After all, this is embarrassing stuff.

Judging from the questions that come up, boys are just as curious as girls about what's happening to their bodies. For every question about menstrual periods or developing breasts, there's one about wet dreams, ejaculations, or hair growth, things like, "How much of that white stuff comes out when a guy comes?" and "When will I grow a beard and start to look like my dad?" Here's one that I got earlier this year:

I am growing a mustash. Not a big mustash, but tiny hares. How can a boy by the age of eleven? He didn't have puberty yet.

The spelling and syntax are unusual, but the spirit behind the question isn't. This boy was worried about the fact that he was developing some fine hairs on his upper lip but he'd never "had puberty," by which he meant that he hadn't ever ejaculated. Generally, facial hair doesn't appear until the sex organs have started to develop, the boy's begun making sperm in his testicles, and he's already begun to ejaculate. But boys develop in different ways, and although it's *unusual* to develop a mustache before these other changes have begun to occur, it's certainly not *abnormal*. This boy, like most young boys, was simply looking for reassurance that what was happening to him was completely normal. It seems little enough to ask.

One reason why parents don't talk to their sons about puberty is undoubtedly simple ignorance. Most fathers didn't get much information from their own fathers. They don't exactly have a storehouse of knowledge to pass on to their sons. Although they have a general idea of what happens during puberty, having gone through it themselves, it's a rare father who can explain to his son exactly why he might have wet dreams or tell him the average age at which a boy first ejaculates. Mothers are at even more of a loss in this respect. They might feel confident enough to make a stab at telling a daughter about menstruation; after all, they've been menstruating themselves for most of their lives. But when it comes to spontaneous erections, wet dreams, and such, they're generally completely at sea.

Another factor in most parents' failure to tell their sons about the body changes of puberty is embarrassment. Sexuality is a difficult, even nigh on to impossible topic for many parents. Even those of us who feel fairly easy about discussing sex may find that there are certain areas of sexuality that we're not entirely comfortable talking over with our children. Take masturbation, for example. It's pretty difficult to discuss puberty with a boy without talking about masturbation; over 90 percent of boys masturbate during puberty. Yet masturbation is a delicate subject, and most of us are bound to feel a little embarrassed discussing it. For one thing, how in the world do you even broach the subject in the first place? What do you say? "Hi, son, been masturbating lately?"

As you may have guessed, I'm coming around to the why-I-wrote-the-book part of this introduction. The purpose of the book is, of course, to provide the basic information that young boys want and need about what's happening to their bodies as they go through puberty, information that we as parents all too often don't have available to give them. Beyond providing the basic facts, I hope that the book will help parents and sons get past the "embarrassment barrier." Ideally, I imagine parents (both the father and the mother) sitting down and reading the book with their sons. Somehow, having the facts printed on a page makes it less embarrassing—someone else is saying it, not *you*; you're just reading the information.

Of course, it's not necessary for both parents to read the book with their son. Either one parent or the other may choose to do so, or it may work better in your particular situation for you to simply give the book to your son to read on his own. You may not even have to give it to him. A number of parents who've read my book about girls and puberty, *What's Happening to My Body? Book for Girls: A Growing Up Guide for Parents and Daughters*, have told me that they bought the book intending to read it with their daughters. But before they'd gotten around to giving it to them, the girls had found the book lying around the house and were already halfway through it.

Regardless of whether you read it separately or together, I hope you'll find a way to talk together about the subjects covered in the book. However, you should be prepared for the fact that, even after your son has read the book, talking it over with him may not be the easiest thing to do. If you come at it head-on by asking a direct question like, "What did you think of the book?" or "Is there anything in the book you'd like to talk about?", it's possible that you'll get a wonderfully detailed critical appraisal of the book, or a series of open, frank questions. What's more likely, though, is that you'll get something along the lines of, "It was okay," or "Naw, there's nothin' I want to know," or "I don-wanna talk about that stuff."

In my experience, it's better to take a slightly different approach. One thing that often works well is for the parent to start things off by saying something along these lines:

"Gee, when I was about your age, I _____."
(Fill in the blank: "noticed my first hairs," "had my first wet dream," "ejaculated for the first time," or whatever.)
"I felt really _____ _____ ."
("Nervous," "excited," "proud," "embarrassed," "afraid," or whatever.)
"In fact, what happened to me was that I ____ _____
_____ ." (Again, fill in the blank with a story about something from your own adolescence, the more embarrassing or stupid the story, the better.)

By using this approach, you make it easier for your kid to open up. By virtue of whatever embarrassing, dumb story you've told about yourself, you've let your kid know that it's okay to be uncertain and less than all-knowingly perfect about the whole business. At least the kids in my class always seem to open up when I tell them about things like:

- The time I got my menstrual period without knowing it and walked around school half the day with a big red blotch on my skirt before anyone told me, and how after that I was sure I could never face going back to school again in my whole life.
- Or the time I bet my best friend, Georgia, my entire allowance that the way people had babies was: the man kissed the woman; a seed from his belly came up his throat, went into her mouth and down her throat, landing in her belly; and nine months later, a baby came out of her belly button. I lost my entire allowance to Georgia.
- Or the time my brother ran for class president and had to give a speech in the auditorium in front of everyone in the whole school, and got a spontaneous erection and didn't know if everyone was laughing at the jokes in his speech or the fact that he had a hard-on.

You get the idea.

Here's another pearl of wisdom: avoid having one all-purpose-ful "talk." It won't fill the bill, no matter how hard you try. It's also better to approach things casually, bringing up the topic from time to time when it seems natural to do so. When I was beginning puberty, my mother sat me down one day to have the Talk. I'm sure she must have explained things in a fairly comprehensible way. All I recall, though, was my mother being horribly nervous and embarrassed and saying a lot of stuff about blood and babies. Then she said something about how when it happened to me, I could come and get some napkins out of the bottom drawer of her bedroom dresser. I remember wondering why in the world she'd be keeping napkins in the bottom drawer of her dresser instead of the top drawer of the kitchen cabinet, which was where napkins were normally kept in our house. But my mother was acting so weird that it just didn't seem like the kind of question to ask at the time. In my experience, a more casual, spur-of-the-moment approach to talking to your child about puberty works better.

Yet another piece of advice: if talking about puberty and sexuality is difficult or embarrassing for you, say so. There's nothing wrong with telling your child, "This is really embarrassing for me. . .," or "My parents never talked to me about this stuff, so I feel kind of weird trying to talk to you. . .," or whatever. Your child is going to pick up on your embarrassment anyway from your tone of voice, your body language, or any one of the other ways we have of communicating what we're really feeling. By trying to pretend you're not uncomfortable, you'll only succeed in confusing your child. Once you've admitted your feelings, you've cleared the air. Your child may adopt a maddeningly smug attitude or be patronizingly sympathetic about your embarrassment, but in the end this is preferable to having him think that there is something weird about the topic itself, that it's not quite right to talk about it.

At this point I must say something about the question that parents most often ask: At what age should you tell your kids about these things? Conventional wisdom holds that you wait until the kids start asking questions. Like many bits of conventional wisdom, this strikes me as a piece of utter nonsense. We don't wait until our kids ask before we teach them how to cross the street safely. Or, if we're religious people, we don't wait until they ask about God before we give them religious instruction. Nor should we wait until they ask before we talk to them about puberty and sex. For one thing, we might end up waiting forever. Kids, having been the recipients of endless unsolicited parental guidance about virtually everything else in their lives, are not very likely to come asking questions about the one area we've been so studiously avoiding. The very fact of our silence on the topic of sexuality sends our kids the message that this is something that it's not okay to talk about.

To my mind, sex education should begin when our children are toddlers. This is not to suggest that you should provide your three-year-old with a sex manual describing sixty-eight different positions for intercourse, or bog down young minds with a detailed explanation of the hormones that initiate and regulate puberty. But once your child reaches the bedtime-story stage, it seems altogether appropriate to introduce the topics of conception, birth, sexuality, and puberty by means of any of the many fine children's picture books that deal with these topics. (Some of my favorites are listed in For Further Reading at the back of this book.)

The book you have here was designed for boys in the nine- to fifteen-year-old group, although it may be appropriate for younger or older boys as well. If sex and related topics are subjects you've been discussing with your child all along, I think you'll find this book is a good bridge between the picture books for younger kids and the publications available for older teens (again, some of my favorite books for older teens are listed in For Further Reading). If this book is your first foray into the sex education of your child, I think that you'll find it an excellent starting place.

I hope the book is one that you'll reread with your son time and again as he's growing older, or that you'll keep around the house so that he can go back to it. What a child of eight or nine takes away from this book will be different from what a boy of thirteen or fourteen does. For example, Chapter 5 deals with spontaneous erections, ejaculations, wet dreams, and masturbation. In my experience, boys of nine or ten are quite curious about these topics, even though most don't actually have their first wet dreams and ejaculations until they are thirteen, fourteen, or older. In fact, younger boys are often more open and easy about discussing these topics than they will be a few years later, when they are experiencing them. At nine or ten, a boy may read Chapter 5 and take away a certain understanding; but at age thirteen or fourteen, when these things are much more real and immediate, the information will be meaningful in different ways. It's important that a boy be prepared for the pubertal changes described in the first five chapters of this book before they happen, but it's also important that he be able to go back and reread the information after these changes have started to take place in his own body.

Chapter 6 deals with girls and puberty. I think it's a good idea for younger boys to have this kind of information. But it will be seen in a different light and taken in by the boy in a more meaningful way once his female classmates have actually begun to go through these changes. So here again, it's important that your boy have this information to go back to as he grows older.

As a parent, you may find that you have some concerns about some of the material covered in this book. Some of the topics, especially those touched upon in Chapter 7, are very controversial. When controversial questions come up in class, I try to present the various points of view and explain why people have them. I think I do a pretty good job of being objective. But sometimes my own point of view comes through. For instance, when discussing masturbation, I explain that some people feel it is wrong or sinful and not at all a good thing to do, and I talk about why they feel that way. But the truth of the matter is that I feel very strongly that masturbation is a perfectly fine, perfectly normal thing to do, and I'm sure that this comes through in what I've written. You may find that your opinions on masturbation or some of the other topics covered in this book are different from mine, but this doesn't mean you have to "throw the baby out with the bath water," as the expression goes. Instead, you can use these differences as an opportunity to explain and elucidate your own attitudes and values to your child.

Regardless of how you decide to deal with the topics of puberty and sexuality or how you decide to use this book, I hope that it will help you and your child to gain a greater understanding of the process of puberty and that it will bring the two of you closer together.

ADDENDUM TO THE NEW EDITION

This book was first published in 1984. I revised and expanded the information three years later in response to the crucial issues raised by the AIDS epidemic, and the growing demand from parents and teachers for earlier and more extensive puberty and sex education for our youngsters.

The first six chapters of this book, the ones that deal with the changes that are happening in children's bodies during puberty, are quite similar to those in the first edition. I haven't made any major revisions in these chapters because there simply wasn't any reason to do so, and I don't expect there ever will be. No matter how much the times may change, kids will undoubtedly continue to go through the same sequence of physical changes, and have the same questions, concerns, and anxieties about these changes generation after generation.

Thus, the major revisions in this new edition come later in the book. The original Chapter 7, which was a sort of catch-all chapter entitled "Sexuality, " has been replaced with three new chapters: "Sexual Intercourse, Pregnancy and Childbirth, and Birth Control"; "Sexually Transmitted Diseases, AIDS, and Other Sexual Health Issues"; and "Romantic and Sexual Feelings." I decided to go into more detail on the subjects I'd only briefly mentioned in the original chapter for two reasons. First, I wasn't entirely satisfied with the original material; it was too sketchy. Indeed, in some cases, it seemed to raise more questions than it answered. Second, parents have encouraged me to go into greater detail about contraception, sexually transmitted diseases (in particular, AIDS), sexual decision-making, and other such topics. Some of these parents told me that they wanted to discuss these issues with their kids, but they weren't exactly certain what to say or how to say it. Others explained that they weren't sure just *how much* to say or *when* (i.e., at what ages) to say it. Some said they'd looked for books that would discuss these subjects in more detail, but either they couldn't find one they liked, or the ones they liked were aimed at older teens. So parents, and teachers as well, urged me to write on these topics in a manner and style appropriate to my readership, that is, for kids in the nine- to fifteen-year-old age group.

Though I was flattered by such requests, I had some serious reservations about expanding the book in this way. I am disturbed by the tendency on the part of parents and educators to give kids *sex* education without first providing them with *puberty* education. It may sound like I'm splitting hairs here, but in my opinion puberty education and sex education are, or at least should be, distinct and separate things. There are, of course, areas of overlap between the two, but basically puberty education focuses on the physical and emotional changes that happen during puberty, while sex education focuses more on intercourse, contraception, the dangers of AIDS, rules for sexual conduct, and so forth.

In the wake of the teen pregnancy and AIDS epidemics, educators and parents are anxious to provide kids with more sex education and to start that education at younger ages than ever before. Schools all across the country have initiated "Just Say No" sex-ed programs (modeled after the drug abuse prevention programs) for seventh graders. The Surgeon General himself has recently suggested that AIDS education begin as early as the third grade.

I suppose that, as someone who's been teaching in this underfunded, largely ignored, and even vilified field for the past ten years, I should be elated over this new enthusiasm and increased funding for sex education. But I'm not, for the fact of the matter is that less than two percent of seventh graders are sexually active, and the vast majority of third-graders are hardly at risk of developing AIDS. There is, no doubt, something to be said for beginning prevention programs early on. But I can't help feeling that much of this new push for more extensive and earlier sex education is more a reflection of adult anxieties about AIDS and adolescent sexual activity than it is a true concern with and understanding of the needs of children.

Elementary school children and seventh-graders don't need *sex* education, they need *puberty* education. Kids of this age have a multitude of questions and fears about the changes that are, or soon will be, taking place in their bodies. I get hundreds and hundreds of letters from kids, the envelopes covered with underscored pleas—"Help!", "URGENT!", "Open At Once!", "Please!

Please! Write Back Right Away!!!''—and inside there'll be five-page letters with intricate diagrams and lengthy explanations of some lump or bump or imagined physical abnormality that has the poor kid worried sick. These children need reassuring puberty education before they're ready for sex education.

When parents and schools ignore puberty education, which addresses the true agendas of children, in favor of sex education, which is more apt to address the agendas of nervous adults, they are, in my opinion, missing the proverbial boat. Kids who aren't given reassuring puberty education when they need it do not respond as well to their parents' or schools' efforts to impart moral codes or even just safe, sane guidelines for sexual conduct.

I think it works something like this: Kids figure, "You were too embarrassed, too busy, too hung up on your own anxiety about my possible sexual activity to respond to my needs for information and reassurance about my changing body. Now, here you are, all freaked out about what I might be doing, trying to push your moral rules and sexual do's and don'ts at me. Well, you're too late. My sexuality is no longer any business of yours. I'm not going to listen to a word you say. So there."

When, on the other hand, kids are given puberty education, the dynamic is altogether different. It's been my experience that kids are enormously grateful for the reassurance they get from such education. I actually have had classes where kids burst into spontaneous applause when I walked into the room. I also have a file drawer full of touching letters from readers thanking me for having allayed some fear or doubt of theirs. Not only are kids grateful when their needs for reassurance are met in this way, but they also develop a profound respect for and trust in the source of that reassurance. Indeed, sometimes the wholesale nature of their trust is a bit unnerving, and I am not always entirely comfortable with the influence I seem to have, especially in situations that involve kids coming to me or writing to me for advice about whether they should become sexually active or how to handle an unplanned pregnancy.

But the point here is that parents need to realize they can forge a very powerful bond with their children if they will "be there" for them during puberty—not to mention how well the ensuing trust and respect will serve all concerned when it comes to later efforts at sex education.

You can see, then, why I had reservations about adding three chapters dealing largely with *sex* education issues to what is, first and foremost, a *puberty* education book. I was afraid that parents would tend to focus on the sex education aspects of the book and ignore the puberty education aspects, the first six chapters.

Obviously, in the end, I did decide (for the reasons described earlier) to go ahead and add these new chapters. But unless your son is already through puberty, please don't let these new chapters become the sole, or even the main, focus of any conversations this book may generate between the two of you. Even if he, himself, tends to gravitate toward talking about the sexual issues, make the effort to steer your conversations back towards the physical and emotional changes of puberty.

Once I'd decided that I would, after all, add these new chapters, I found myself facing certain problems which I think are worth mentioning here. These stemmed from the fact that my readership covers such a wide age range—anywhere from age nine to fifteen, or even older. This wasn't too much of a problem when the book dealt almost exclusively with puberty, but it presented difficulties in the new chapters.

Consider, for example, Chapter 9, which deals with romantic and sexual feelings. Older boys frequently have questions about dating or making decisions about sex, but younger boys are often in the I-could-care-less-about-girls stage. By the same token, issues such as how to handle the fact that your best friend is a girl are usually not very relevant to the lives of most fifteen-year-olds. So, Chapter 9 had to cover a spectrum that began with opposite-sex friendships and stretched all the way to questions about sexual decision-making. I realized that those whose questions fell on one end of the spectrum might not find the questions on the other end very interesting or applicable to their lives. I solved this problem by simply telling readers to skip any sections that didn't interest them, and I hope that you will also point this out to your son.

The wide age range was more problematic in the section on birth control in Chapter 7. The kind of contraceptive information that younger boys want or need is usually quite different from the sort of information that might be appropriate for a fifteen-year-old. Birth control isn't a major part of my curriculum for my younger classes, and the topic usually only comes up in response to questions in the class question box. Answering younger kids' questions is generally just a matter of correcting their mistaken ideas. (For example, they often think that taking birth control pills makes a woman infertile forever, and because they heard it called *The Pill*, they think it's about the size of a golf ball.) By and large, the only real interest the nine-year-old boys in my classes have in birth control methods is in seeing if they can make a water balloon out of a condom.

Fifteen-year-olds, on the other hand, may have a much different level of interest and a much greater need for information. Thirty-five percent of the fifteen-year-old boys in this country have had sex; thus, a boy of this age may well need specific, practical contraceptive advice. But he won't find it here.

Detailed, user-oriented birth control information would not only have been way over the heads of many of my readers, but including such information would have lengthened the book to the point where its sheer size alone would have scared off many younger readers. So I made a compromise and, like most compromises, it wasn't entirely satisfactory. The information here is appropriate for most of my readers. Still, there is probably more contraceptive information than a nine-year-old will want or need, and definitely less than a sexually active teen should have. So if you have an older son who is, or may be, sexually active, please don't rely on this book alone to meet his needs. At the very least, you should see that he gets (and reads) one of the books listed in the bibliography. If, on the other hand, you have a younger son (or for that matter a son of any age) who isn't interested in this topic or finds the information "over his head," he can, of course, skip it, although there's certainly no harm done if he were to go ahead and read it.

I know there are some parents who worry that giving kids access to information about birth control will encourage them to go out and experiment sexually. To such parents it seems patently obvious: The greater the availability of birth control, the greater the likelihood of kids having sex. But adolescents' minds work differently, and to them birth control and sexual activity are not necessarily linked. The average teenager is sexually active for at least a year before even considering using a method of birth control. Once they have a method, about two-thirds of them never use it or use it only sporadically. Besides, if birth control were causing teens to be sexually active, we wouldn't have upwards of a million teenage pregnancies each year, and we wouldn't be faced with the alarming statistic that four out of every ten of today's fourteen-year-olds will have been pregnant at least once by the end of their teen years. In the ten years that I've been working with kids, I have only known two (count 'em, *two*) teenagers who obtained a method of birth control *before* they started having sex. If you think teenagers are having sex because of the availability of contraception, you're putting the cart before the horse, at least by adolescents' logic. It just doesn't work that way.

So there is no harm done if your child should read the section on birth control, even though he may be way too young to have a practical need for it. Too many parents wait until their kids have begun dating or going steady to introduce the topic. Their first parent/child contraception conversations often come in the context of a parental message like, "I don't want you having sex yet, but if you do, I want you to use something." I think that's a perfectly legitimate message for a parent to send, but it's an awfully highly charged situation in which to initiate contraception education efforts, and kids are often confused by what sounds to them like a double message. It's much easier, less confusing to kids—and undoubtedly more effective—to begin discussions on birth control earlier.

Writing the section on sexually transmitted diseases in Chapter 8 posed problems similar to the ones I faced with birth control, and I made a similar sort of compromise. Younger readers may find more information than they need, and there may not be enough for sexually active readers. Here again, for the older boys, there are resources listed in the bibliography, and the younger readers can skip overly detailed material.

In my classes for older teens, I am quite frank and detailed, graphic even, in discussing AIDS and *all* the modes of transmission, for as the Surgeon General has so aptly put it, "You can't talk of the dangers of snake poisoning and not mention snakes." But in my classes for younger kids, I do not discuss the specific "high-risk" sex practice that, according to many experts, accounts for the high incidence of AIDS among male homosexuals. I'm not being coy in failing to say precisely which practice I am talking about here. I'm being deliberately obtuse because even younger kids sometimes read the parents' introductions to my books, and I don't think it's appropriate to discuss this high-risk practice with them. First of all, it's not necessary. In my experience, younger children's curiosity is quite satisfied with less specific explanations, and since they don't engage in this practice, there is no need to warn them against it. Second, all my instincts as a teacher tell me that a discussion of this high-risk sexual practice would be far too confusing and upsetting for many younger children.

At any rate, the AIDS discussion in this book is one that, to my mind, is appropriate for younger children. Those of you with older sons will, I hope, make use of the resources listed in the bibliography as well as my newest book, *Lynda Madaras Talks to Teens About AIDS*.

I hope this book will help you and your child develop an even closer and more loving relationship.

CHAPTER 1

Puberty

It was great. I remember thinking, "I'm not just a kid anymore!" I loved it!

John, age 26

It was weird. I was tired all the time and sleeping a whole lot. I wasn't really sure what was happening to me.

Bill, age 19

People make it sound like it's this big dramatic thing that all of a sudden happens one day. It's not like that. It's not like some guy pops up and says, "Hey, kid, this is it. Now it's going to happen to you."

Jackson, age 33

It seemed like I woke up one day and everything had changed. I was a different person in a different body.

Sam, age 35

Even though they had very different things to say about it, all these men are talking about the same thing

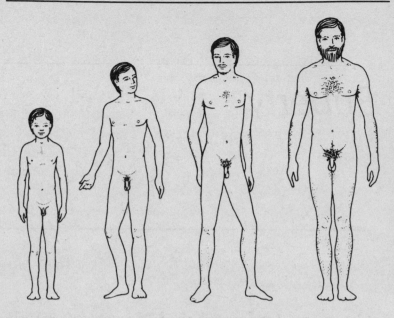

Illustration 1. Male puberty changes. As boys go through puberty, they get taller, their shoulders get wider, their bodies more muscular, their genital organs develop, and they begin to grow hair on their genitals, underarms, faces, chests, arms and legs.

—*puberty*.* Puberty is a time in people's lives when their bodies are changing from children's bodies into adults' bodies. As you can see from Illustration 1, a boy's body changes quite a bit as he goes through puberty. For one thing, he gets taller. Of course, we grow taller all through childhood. But during puberty, a boy grows taller at a faster rate than he ever will again in his

* *puberty* (PEW-bur-tee)   The word puberty is pronounced with the accent on the first part of the word, PEW. You say this part of the word loudest, with the most emphasis. Throughout this book, there are a number of words that you may not have heard before. Whenever we use one of these words for the first time, we have included a pronunciation guide like this at the bottom of the page.

life. During this growth spurt, he may gain as many as four or more inches in one year.

The general shape of his body changes too, so that his shoulders become broader and his hips seem narrower in comparison. His muscles develop and his body strength increases. His whole body begins to look more "manly." Hair grows in places where it never grew before—around his penis, under his arms, and on his face. His penis and his scrotum, the sac of skin just beneath his penis, get bigger. At the same time that these changes are happening on the outside of his body, other changes are taking place on the inside of his body.

For some boys, these changes happen so fast that they seem to take place overnight. But they don't really happen that quickly. Puberty happens slowly and gradually, over a period of months or years. These changes may start when a boy is as young as ten. Or they may not happen until he is fifteen or older. Regardless of when they start for you, you'll probably have a lot of questions about what is happening to your body. We hope this book will answer at least some of those questions.

"We" are my friend Dane and I. The two of us worked together to make this book. About a year before I wrote this book, my daughter, Area, and I wrote another book, a lot like this one, about how puberty happens in girls' bodies. (It's called *The What's Happening to my Body? Book for Girls.*)

Even though I'm a medical writer, and I teach classes about puberty and know quite a lot of scientific facts about puberty, I thought it would be a good idea to

penis (PEE-niss)
scrotum (SKRO-tum)

get my daughter's help in writing the girl's book. She was going through puberty herself at the time. Of course, I had been through puberty too, but it was a long time ago. I was thirty-six when Area and I wrote the girl's book, and to tell you the truth, I wasn't really sure I could think back across all those years and remember the kinds of feelings and questions I had back then. I figured Area could give me the kid's point of view on things. So I talked her into writing the girl's book with me, and I guess we did a pretty good job because Esther Margolis, the woman who published the girl's book, said, "Why don't you do a book about boys and puberty?"

I thought that sounded like a good idea, but once again, I wanted to get the kid's point of view. It seemed especially important for this book because I'm a woman, and I don't have firsthand knowledge of how puberty happens in a boy's body. The trouble was that I don't have a son. So I decided to find a boy that I knew really well and who felt comfortable enough with me and with himself to work on a book like this. That's when I thought of Dane. Dane's mom, Katie, and I have been good friends for years and years, and I've known Dane ever since he barely came up to my knees. (He's way past my knees now. In fact, he's eighteen and six feet tall and I have to stick my nose up in the air when I want to talk to him.)

Dane thought the idea of doing this book sounded good too, so he agreed to provide the kid's point of view. He read over the various parts of the book and told me when I'd written something really dumb or when I'd forgotten to explain something or when what I'd said was confusing or unclear. And we both talked to lots of men and boys to find out what happened to *them* during puberty, how they felt about it, and what kinds of questions and concerns they had at the time. You'll hear their voices throughout this book. Some of the quotes we've used are from kids in my classes.* During the school year, I teach a class in puberty at Sequoyah School in Pasadena, California. The kids in my classes and the men and boys Dane and I talked to had a lot of questions and a lot of things to say about puberty. So, in a sense, they too helped write this book.

Way back when I first started teaching classes about puberty, I decided that the best way to begin was to talk about how babies are made, because the changes that happen in our bodies during puberty happen because we are getting ready for a time when we may decide to make babies.

I didn't think I'd have any big problems in teaching the class. "Nothing to it," I told myself. "I'll just go on in there and start by talking to the kids about how babies are made. Probably I'll have to draw some pictures on the blackboard to help explain things, and maybe I don't draw really well, but we'll manage."

"No problem," I told myself.

Boy, was I wrong! I'd hardly even opened my mouth before everyone, or almost everyone, in the class started acting crazy. Kids were giggling and nudging one another and getting all red in the face. One boy even fell off his chair. People were acting all sorts of strange ways because, in order to talk about how babies are made, I had to talk about *sex*, and sex, as you may have noticed, is a *very big deal*. Kids—and, in fact, people of all ages—often act embarrassed, giggly, or secretive when the topic of sex comes up.

---

* We changed the names of the boys and men we quoted in this book in order not to embarrass them after they'd been generous enough to share their feelings and thoughts about puberty with us.

Even the word itself is confusing because *sex* can mean so many different things and is used in so many different ways. In the simplest meaning of the word, *sex* refers to the different kinds of bodies that men and women have. There are a lot of differences between male and female bodies, but one of the most obvious is that a male has a penis and a scrotum, and a female has a vulva and a vagina. These body parts, or organs (*organ* is another word for body part), are called *sex organs*. People belong to either the male sex or the female sex, depending on which type of sex organs they have.

The word *sex* is also used in other ways. We may say that two people are "having sex." Having sex, or having *sexual intercourse*, involves a man putting his penis into a woman's vagina. Or we may say that two people are "being sexual with each other," which means that they are having sexual intercourse or that they are holding, touching, or caressing each other's sexual organs. We may say that we are "feeling sexual," which means that we are having feelings or thoughts about our sexual organs, about being sexual with another person, or about having sexual intercourse.

Our sex organs are very private parts of our bodies. We usually keep them covered up, and we don't talk about them in public very often. Having sex, being sexual with someone, or having sexual feelings are also private matters that don't get talked about very often. I suppose that if I'd had half a brain in my head, I would have realized that coming into a classroom and talking about sex and penises and vaginas and making

vulva (VUL-va)
vagina (vah-JIE-nah)
intercourse (IN-ter-korse)

babies and all that stuff that people don't usually talk about was going to cause a big commotion.

After that first class, though, I caught on. I decided that if we were going to get all silly and giggly when we talked about these things in class, we might as well get *really* silly and giggly. So now I start the first class of the year by giving everyone photocopies of the two drawings you see in Illustration 2 and red and blue colored pencils that we use to color the drawings.

THE SEX ORGANS

Illustration 2 shows the female and male sex organs, also called the *genitals* or *genital organs*. Everyone has sex organs on both the inside and outside of the body, and they change as we go through puberty. These pictures show how the sex organs on the outside of the body look in grown men and women.

Nowadays, I start my puberty classes by holding up the picture of the male sex organs. I explain to the class that the sex organs on the outside of a man's body have two main parts and that the scientific names for these parts are the *penis* and the *scrotum*. When I pass out the drawings and start talking about the penis and the scrotum, the kids in my class still giggle like mad, nudge one another, or fall off their chairs in embarrassment, but I don't pay much attention to all of this. I simply say, "Okay, the penis itself also has two parts: the *shaft* and the *glans*. Find the shaft of the penis on your drawing and color it with blue and red stripes." Some kids keep giggling and some get very serious about the coloring, but they all start coloring. Why don't you color

genitals (JEN-a-tulls)
glans (GLANZ)

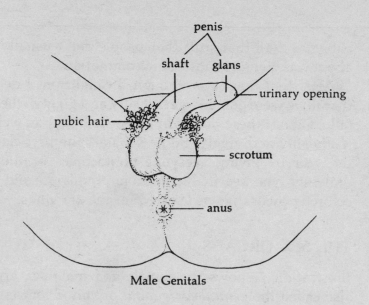

Male Genitals

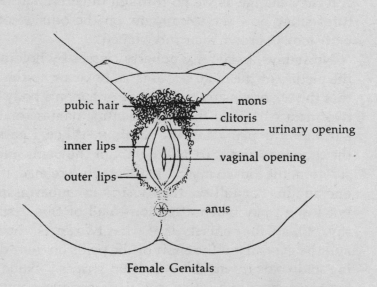

Female Genitals

Illustration 2. Male and female genitals

the shaft in, too. (Unless, of course, this book belongs to someone else or to a library. One of the people we admire most in the world is a wonderful lady named Lou Ann Sobieski. She's a librarian, and Dane and I would be in *very hot water* if Lou Ann thought we were telling people to color on library books.)

The glans, or head, of the penis has a ridge of skin around the lower part called the *corona*, and after the class has colored the shaft, I tell them to color the corona red.

After they've colored the corona, I ask the class to find the small slit at the tip of the penis and color it red. This is the *urinary opening*, the opening through which urine (pee) leaves the body. There's usually a bit less giggling by now as they start coloring the urinary opening, because it's smaller and they have to pay more attention to what they are doing. Next, we color in the glans itself. I usually recommend blue, but color it any way you want, just as long as it's colored differently from the other parts so that it will stand out clearly.

The *scrotum* is a loose bag of skin that lies beneath the penis. Another name for the scrotum is the scrotal sac. Inside the scrotum are two egg-shaped organs called *testes* or *testicles*. You can't see them in these pictures, but I like to mention them at this point because they have a lot to do with making babies. (We'll talk more about them in the following pages.)

corona (ko-RO-na)
urinary (YUR-in-airee)
urine (YUR-in)
testes (TES-teez)
testicles (TES-ti-kuls)

I also explain that the curly hairs they see growing around the genitals have a special name. These hairs are called *pubic hairs*, and I ask the class to color them too.

Finally, we come to the *anus*. The anus is the opening through which feces or bowel movements leave our bodies. It's not really a sex organ, but because it is located in the genital area, I like to mention it.

By the time we've colored in the different parts, I've said the word *penis* in front of the class about twenty-eight times, so everyone gets used to my saying this word that usually doesn't get said out loud in classrooms (or anywhere else for that matter), and they no longer have to get all crazy and giggly each time I use it. Besides that, the pictures look so funny that everyone gets to laughing out loud, and that makes it easier for all of us to deal with the nervousness that most of us feel when we talk about sex organs.

I also have another reason for getting the kids in my class to color in these drawings: I think it helps them to learn the names of these organs. If you just look at the drawing and see that this part is labeled the *penis* and that part the *scrotum*, it's all kind of jumbled and doesn't stick in your mind. But if you spend a few moments coloring them in, you have to pay attention and you'll remember better. These are important parts of the body, so it's worth the effort. If this book isn't yours and you can't color in it, try making a tracing of these drawings and coloring on the tracing.

While we're going through the business of coloring the drawings, we also talk about slang words. As you know, people don't always use the scientific names for

pubic (PEW-bic)
anus (AY-nus)
feces (FEE-sees)
bowel (BOW-ul)

these body parts. Mostly they use slang words. I've found that if we don't talk about these words right out loud in class, kids are always leaning over and whispering them to one another and giggling madly and acting crazy again. So while we're coloring our drawings, all of the kids yell out the slang words they've heard for penis, scrotum, and testicles and I make a list of them on the blackboard. Here are some of the words that we've come up with:

SLANG WORDS FOR THE PENIS, SCROTUM, AND TESTICLES

PENIS			SCROTUM AND TESTICLES	
cock	peter	tool	balls	cujones
dick	rod	frankfurter	nuts	things
prick	dingus	thing	eggs	bangers
schlong	dork	banger	rocks	hangers
wee-wee	meat	dinky	jewels	stones
wanger	pisser	penie	cubes	seeds
pecker	hot dog	weenie	sac	bag
wang	weiner	dong		

As I explain to the kids in my class, I personally don't object to using slang words to refer to sex organs. In fact, I think that they are sometimes easier to use and they make people more comfortable about talking about these body parts. But some people do object to these slang words, and they may get upset if they hear you using them. You may or may not care about upsetting people in this way, but you should at least be aware that there are people who find slang words offensive.

Next, I usually show my class a picture like the one in Illustration 3 and explain about circumcision.

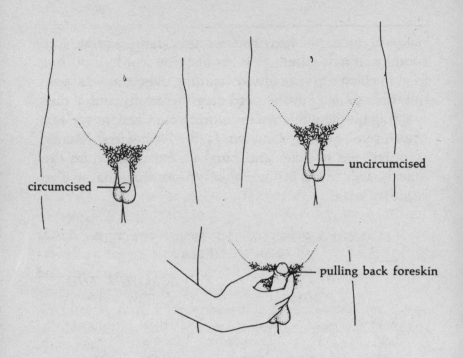

Illustration 3. Circumcision

Circumcision is an operation in which the doctor cuts away a fold of skin called the *foreskin* from around the top of the penis. The foreskin covers the glans of the penis, but it can be pulled down the shaft, as shown in Illustration 3. In this country, most circumcisions are done when babies are two or three days old. The foreskin is pulled up over the top of the penis and a special instrument is used to cut the foreskin away. Not all parents choose to have their babies circumcised. If you have not been circumcised, it is important that you pull the foreskin back and clean under it whenever you bathe or shower, because a secretion called smegma

circumcision (sir-cum-SISH-un)
circumcised (sir-cum-SIZED)
smegma (SMEG-ma)

collects under the foreskin and can cause an unpleasant odor or irritation.

One of the first questions that the kids in my class ask when I talk about this subject is, "Why do people have their babies circumcised?" Sometimes it is done for religious reasons. It is a custom in the Jewish and Muslim religions for parents to circumcise their boys. Until recently, most boys in this country were circumcised even if their parents were not Jewish or Muslim. Doctors encouraged circumcision because it makes it easier to clean the penis, because they felt the foreskin could trap germs and the boy could be more likely to get an infection, and because it was thought that uncircumcised men were more likely to get cancer of the penis. But as long as a boy pulls the foreskin back and cleans the glans of the penis regularly, he isn't any more likely to get infections than someone who has been circumcised. Moreover, doctors are no longer certain that being circumcised really has anything to do with how likely it is that a man will get cancer of the penis. Besides, cancer of the penis is a rare disease. (Boys, by the way, *never* get cancer of the penis. It only happens to men, usually only to men over the age of fifty.) Because of all this, many doctors and parents are wondering whether it is really worth it to put a newborn baby through the pain and discomfort of circumcision. In the past ten years or so, more and more parents have been deciding not to have their male babies circumcised.

As we said, the operation is usually done when the baby is two or three days old. Occasionally, though, a boy or man who wasn't circumcised at birth may decide to have the operation done later on. Often this is because his foreskin is too tight or is stuck to the head of the penis and cannot be fully rolled down the shaft. This can cause swelling and pain, and circumcision is often the best solution. But these problems are very rare. It is unusual for an older boy or man to have the circumcision operation. If you haven't been circumcised at birth, you probably never will be.

The only difference between circumcised and uncircumcised males is that circumcised males don't have a foreskin. Otherwise, their penis looks, feels, and works the same way.

When we have finished coloring the male sex organs, we move on to the female sex organs shown in Illustration 2. The genital organs on the outside of a woman's body are sometimes referred to as the *vulva*. The vulva has many parts. We usually start at the top with the fleshy mound called the *mons*, which, in grown women, is covered with crisp, curly pubic hairs. Color the mons and the pubic hair blue. Then we move toward the bottom of the mons where it divides into two folds or flaps of skin called the *outer lips*. Try coloring these with red stripes. In between the outer lips lie the *inner lips*—blue stripes for the inner lips. The inner lips join together at the top, where there is a small, bud-shaped organ called the *clitoris*. Color it red. Just down from the clitoris is the woman's urinary opening, through which urine leaves the body. Color it blue. Below the urinary opening is another opening called the *vaginal opening*. It leads into a hollow pouch or cavity inside the body called the *vagina*. Use your imagination—color it red, blue, striped, polka-dot, or whatever.

You may have heard people use the word *vagina* to refer to the vulva. Actually, the vagina is *inside* the body. The vulva, which includes the lips, the clitoris, and the urinary and vaginal openings, is on the outside

mons (MONZ)
clitoris (KLIT-or-iss)
vaginal (VAH-jin-ul)

of the body. It is not really correct to mix these terms up, but people do it all the time.

Finally, we come to the *anus*. Color it as well.

While we're coloring in the female genitals, we also make a list of slang words used to refer to these parts of a woman's body.

SLANG WORDS FOR THE CLITORIS,
VULVA, AND VAGINA

CLITORIS	*VULVA AND VAGINA*		
clit	cunt	box	snatch
bud	pussy	beaver	poontang
pea	muff	honeypot	pudie
man in the boat	stuff	hole	slit

By the time we've finished coloring both these pictures, everyone has giggled off a good deal of embarrassment. The kids have also gotten a pretty good idea of where these body parts are, which makes it a lot easier to understand how a man and a woman make babies.

SEXUAL INTERCOURSE

In order to make a baby, a man and a woman must have sexual intercourse. When I tell the kids in my class about this, they usually have two questions. One thing they want to know is how a man's penis could get into a woman's vagina. I explain that sometimes the penis gets stiff and hard and stands out from the body, as shown in Illustration 4. This is called an *erection*, and it can happen when a male is feeling sexual or is having sex with someone, and at other times too. The inside of the

erection (e-REK-shun)

penis is made up of spongy tissue. When a male is having an erection, special blood passageways in this spongy tissue fill up with blood, which makes the penis get bigger and harder and stand out from the body. Some people call an erection a "boner" or a "hard-on" because the penis feels so stiff and hard. It's almost as if there really is a bone in there. But there isn't any bone, just blood-filled, spongy tissue.

While it is erect, the penis can slide right into the vaginal opening. The vaginal opening isn't very large, but it's very elastic and stretchy, so the erect penis can easily fit in there.

In addition to wanting to know *how,* some of the kids in my classes want to know *why* in the world anyone would want to do this.

A man and a woman have sexual intercourse for all sorts of reasons. It is a special way of being close with

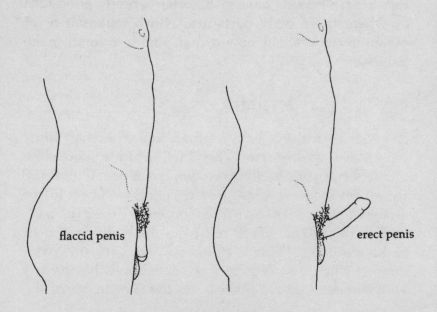

flaccid penis   erect penis

Illustration 4. Erection

another person. It also feels good, which some of the kids in my class find hard to believe. But the sex organs have many nerve endings. If these parts of our bodies are stroked or rubbed in the right ways, the nerve endings send messages to pleasure centers in our brains, and we get pleasurable feelings all over our bodies. People also have sexual intercourse because they want to have a baby, but babies don't start to grow every time a man and a woman have intercourse, just sometimes.

MAKING BABIES

In order to make a baby, two things are needed: an *ovum* from a woman's body and a *sperm* from a man's body. You may have heard adults talking about an ovum and calling it "a woman's egg" or talking about a sperm and calling it "a man's seed." When many of the kids in my classes hear the word *egg*, they think about the kind of eggs that chickens lay and that we buy at grocery stores to scramble up for breakfast. When they hear the word *seed*, they think about the things we plant in the ground in order to grow flowers or vegetables. But the ovum and the sperm are not like these kinds of eggs and seeds. For one thing, an ovum is much smaller than the eggs we cook up for breakfast—in fact, it is much smaller than the smallest dot you could make with the tip of even the sharpest pencil point. And a sperm is even smaller than an ovum.

I think the best way to think of a sperm and an ovum is to think of each of them as being half of a seed. When these two halves of a seed come together, a human baby begins to grow.

ovum (OH-vum)
sperm (SPURM)

Sperm are made in the testicles, the two egg-shaped organs inside the scrotum. Sometimes, when a man and a woman are having sexual intercourse, and the man's penis is inside the woman's vagina, a man *ejaculates*. When a man ejaculates, the muscles of the penis contract, and the sperm are pumped out of the testicles, through the *urethra* (the hollow tube in the center of the penis), and out the opening in the center of the glans, as shown in Illustration 5. A teaspoonful or so of a creamy fluid, called *semen*, full of millions of tiny, microscopic sperm, comes out of the penis. This liquid is also called "ejaculate," or in slang terms "come" or "jism."

After the sperm leave the penis, they start swimming up toward the top of the vagina. They pass through a tiny opening at the top of the vagina that leads into an organ called the *uterus* (see Illustration 6). The uterus is a hollow organ, and, in a grown woman, it is only about the size of a clenched fist. But the thick muscular walls of the uterus are quite elastic, and, like a balloon, the uterus can expand to many times its size. The uterus has to be able to expand like this because it is here, inside a woman's uterus, that a baby grows.

Some of the sperm swim up to the top of the uterus and into one of two little tubes or tunnels called the *fallopian tubes*. Not all the sperm make it this far. Some drift back down to the uterus and out into the vagina, where they join other sperm that never made it out of the vagina. These sperm and the rest of the creamy, white liquid dribble back down the vagina and out of the woman's body.

Women, too, make seeds in their bodies. When we

ejaculates (e-JACK-you-lates)
urethra (YUR-ee-thra)
semen (SEE-men)

ejaculate (e-JACK-you-lat)
uterus (YOU-ter-us)
fallopian (fuh-LOPE-e-an)

 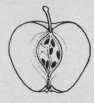

If you cut an apple in half, you would be able to see the seeds and core on the inside of the apple. This drawing, which shows the inside of an apple, is called a cross section.

The drawing below is also a cross section. It shows the inside of the penis and scrotum.

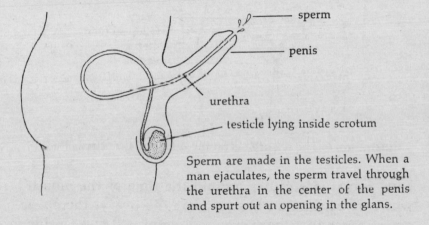

Sperm are made in the testicles. When a man ejaculates, the sperm travel through the urethra in the center of the penis and spurt out an opening in the glans.

Illustration 5. Ejaculation

are talking about just one of these seeds, we use the word *ovum*. When we are talking about more than one, we use the word *ova*. The ova ripen inside two little organs called *ovaries*. In a mature girl, the ovaries produce a ripe seed about once a month. When this seed is ripe, it leaves the ovary and travels down the fallopian tube toward the uterus. If a woman and man

ova (OH-vah)
ovaries (OH-vah-reez)

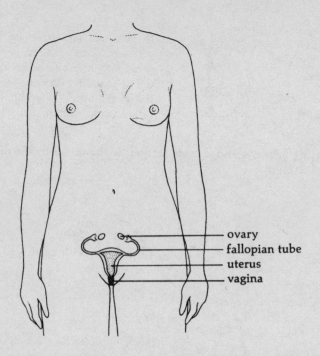

ovary
fallopian tube
uterus
vagina

Illustration 6. The sex organs on the inside of the female body

have sexual intercourse around the time of the month when the ripe ovum has just left the ovary, there's a good chance that the sperm and ovum will meet inside the tube. When a sperm and ovum meet, the sperm penetrates the outer shell of the ovum and moves inside it. This joining together of the ovum and the sperm is called *fertilization*, and when a sperm has penetrated an ovum, we say that the ovum has been fertilized.

Most of the time, the ovum travels through the fallopian tube without meeting up with a sperm, and the tiny ovum just disintegrates. But if the ovum has been fertilized, it doesn't disintegrate. Instead, the fertilized ovum plants itself on one of the inside walls of the uterus, and over the next nine months, it grows into a

fertilization (FUR-till-ih-zay-shun)

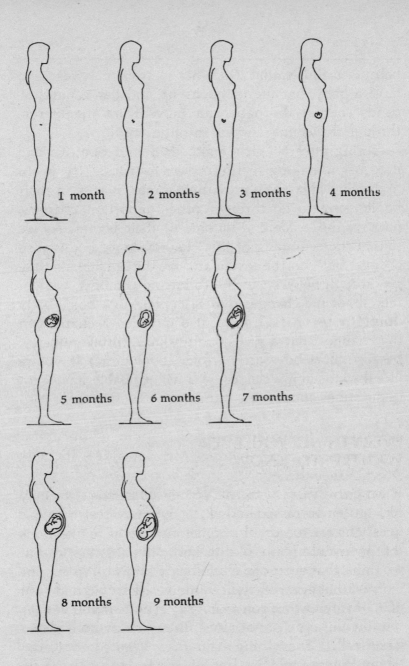

Illustration 7. Stages of pregnancy. A fertilized ovum plants itself on the inside wall of the uterus, and over the next nine months, it develops into a baby.

baby (see Illustration 7). When a woman is ready to have a baby, her uterus opens up and her vagina expands so that the baby can move from the uterus, through the vagina, and out into the world.

During puberty, girls make their first ripe ova and boys begin making sperm in their testicles. Girls begin to develop breasts, to grow hair in new places on their bodies, and to go through other important changes, both on the inside and outside of their bodies. As we said at the beginning of this chapter, boys' bodies also change, both on the inside and on the outside, as they go through puberty. In the following chapters, we will talk about the changes that take place in a boy's body during puberty. (We have also included a chapter on the changes that a girl goes through during puberty, because most boys are curious about girls.) If you're like the kids in my classes, you will probably have a lot of questions about these things.

EVERYTHING YOU EVER
WANTED TO KNOW . . .

It isn't always easy to ask certain questions. We may feel too embarrassed to ask, or we may feel that our questions are too dumb. Sometimes we have questions that we would really like to know the answers to, but we think that everyone else already knows. We may be worried that everyone will think we are stupid and "out of it" if we show we don't know by asking. If you've ever felt like this, you're not alone. In my classes, we play a game called Everything You Ever Wanted to Know About Puberty and Sex but Were Afraid to Ask. I pass out slips of paper at the beginning of each class so that the kids can write down their questions and put them in a special question box. They don't have to sign their names to the questions. I am the only one who gets to see them, so nobody can look at the handwriting and figure out who wrote the question. I also leave the locked question box and some slips of paper somewhere in the classroom so that kids can write down questions whenever one crosses their mind. At the end of each class, I take the questions out of the box, read them out loud, and answer them the best I can.

Here are some of the many kinds of questions that have come up in our question box:

"When will I grow a beard and start to look like my dad?"

"How much of that white stuff comes out of a man's penis when he ejaculates?"

"Why do you sometimes get a hard-on when you're not even thinking about sex?"

"Is there something wrong if you have one testicle lower than the other?"

"Why do you have to wear a jockstrap?"

"What's the largest penis measurement in the world? Can a penis be too small? Will it get bigger when I get older?"

"Which way should your penis curve when it's hard?"

"How come people get pimples when they're going through puberty?"

"What is a wet dream?"

"Can a boy grow breasts?"

"Exactly what does 'jacking off' or 'playing with yourself' mean, and is it okay to do it?"

"I have little white bumps on my penis. Does that mean I have some kind of disease?"

"How do twins and triplets happen? Do they come out at the same time?"

"I have a pain in my penis and some white stuff that looks like milk has been coming out. What's wrong?"

"How old should a person be before they have sex?"

"How long can sperm live?"

"If you ejaculate too often, can this hurt you? Will you run out of sperm?"

"Is it true that girls bleed once a month after they go through puberty?"

In the following pages, we will answer these and other questions that have come up in the question box or that were asked by the boys and men we talked to about puberty. You may find that you have questions that are not answered by this book. If so, perhaps your dad or mom, the school nurse, one of your teachers, or another adult you know can help you find answers to your questions. Friends your own age may be able to answer your questions, but a lot of kids find that the answers they get from other kids are not always right. It is usually better to ask an adult you know and feel comfortable talking to. Or you could write to us. Your envelope should be addressed like this:

> Lynda Madaras
> Newmarket Press
> 18 East 48th Street
> New York, NY 10017

Be sure to include a self-addressed, stamped envelope so we can write back to you.

USING THIS BOOK

You may want to read this book with your parents, with a friend, or all by yourself. You may want to read it straight through from beginning to end, or you may want to jump around, reading a chapter here and there, depending on what you are most curious about. However you decide to go about using this book, we hope that you will enjoy it and that you will learn as much from reading it as we did from writing it.

CHAPTER 2

The Stages of Puberty

Growing vegetables is one of my hobbies. Three or four mornings a week, I'm out there in my garden pulling up weeds or planting things or yelling at the birds, which are always eating up my peas. I like to pretend that my hobby is a very sensible one and that I save lots of money by growing my own vegetables. But this isn't really true. In fact, if you added up all the hours I spend working in my garden and all the money I spend on things like seeds, gardening books, fertilizers, and plastic netting to keep the birds off the peas, each pound of peas I get out of my garden probably costs me about fifty bucks.

You may be asking yourself what in the world my expensive hobby of growing vegetables has to do with boys and puberty. The answer is, nothing at all. Except maybe for this one thing: each of the plants in my garden has its own way and time of growing. I have never been able to figure out why this is so. I can take two seeds from the same package that look exactly alike and plant them in the same row of my garden right next to each other. I will give them both the exact same amount of water, and they will both get the same amount of sunshine. Yet one seedling will come popping out of the ground and grow to a height of three or four inches before the other one has barely even broken through the top layer of soil. Boys, too, seem to have their own way and time of growing. One may start to go through puberty when he is only ten. Another might not start until he is fourteen.

The so-called "average" or "normal" or "regular" age at which boys start to go through puberty is around eleven or twelve. But very few boys are what we call average. The boys you see in Illustration 8 are both twelve years old. Both are completely healthy, normal, regular boys; however, one boy has already developed quite a bit. He has obviously started puberty. He has already gotten quite tall. He has grown a lot of pubic hair. His body has lots of muscles, and his penis and scrotum have grown quite a bit too. The other boy has barely even started to go through the body changes of puberty.

No one is sure why some boys start to go through puberty at a fairly young age and others do not start until they are older. It probably has something to do with a boy's family. If both your mother and father come from families in which people tend to start puberty at an early age, you probably will too. Or if both your parents come from familes in which people do not go through puberty until they are older, then you probably won't start to go through puberty until later too. This is not a hard and fast rule. A boy may be a later starter even if his parents were early starters. The opposite may also be true. But parents and children are

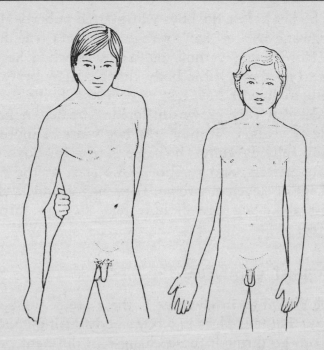

Illustration 8. Two twelve-year-olds. Both these boys are twelve. One has already developed quite a bit. The other hasn't begun to go through the body changes of puberty.

often alike in this way. You might want to ask your mom and dad how old they were when they started puberty.

Once a boy starts to go through the body changes of puberty, he may develop rather quickly or he may develop more slowly. I have noticed that the first seedlings to pop up in my garden always seem to be a step ahead of the other seedlings. They develop into fully grown, ripe plants before the others and are ready to be harvested first. A lot of people think that the same kind of thing holds true for boys going through puberty. They figure that the boys who start early will always be a step ahead of the other boys and will develop grown-up, adult bodies before the boys who started puberty at the average age or later than average. This isn't true, however. How young or how old a boy is when he first starts to go through the body changes of puberty has nothing to do with how fast he develops. Early starters may develop very grown-up looking bodies in just a couple of years, or it may take five years or more for them to fully develop. The same is true for boys who are late starters, and for boys who start at the more usual age of eleven or twelve. They may be quick, slow, or just about average in how fast they go through puberty.

THE FIRST CHANGES

As we explained in Chapter 1, there are a number of changes that take place in a boy's body during puberty. Boys can go through these changes in different order. For some boys, the first change that happens is that they begin to grow pubic hair. For most boys, though, the first change that takes place during puberty is that their sex organs begin to grow. This usually happens before they begin to develop pubic hairs, grow taller, or go through the other changes that take place during puberty. As puberty continues, the sex organs—the penis, scrotum, and testicles—continue to grow larger.

THE FIVE STAGES OF
GENITAL DEVELOPMENT

Doctors have divided the growth and development of the genital, or sex, organs into the five stages shown in Illustration 9. You may be in one of these stages, or you may be in between one stage and another. See if you can find the stage you are closest to.

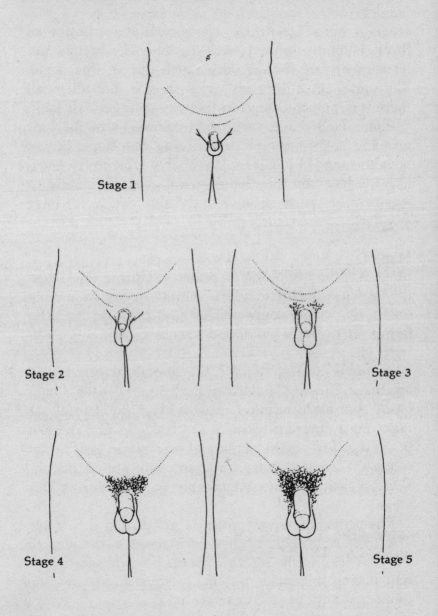

Illustration 9. The five stages of male genital development

Stage 1

Stage 1 starts when you are born and continues all through your childhood years. Your penis, scrotum, and testicles do not change very much during this stage. They may get a little bit larger in size, but all in all there is not much change in the way your genitals look.

Some boys have soft, light-colored, straight hair growing in their genital area during this stage. If you have this kind of hair, it will probably look pretty much like the hair you may have growing on your belly or legs or other parts of your body. But you won't have any dark- colored, curly pubic hair yet.

Stage 2

Stage 2 is the beginning of puberty. During this stage, the testicles get larger and the scrotal sac begins to hang lower. Of course, your testicles have been getting a bit larger all through childhood (Stage 1). But once puberty starts, they grow at a faster rate.

As the testicles get larger, the scrotal sac gets longer and hangs lower. The scrotum also gets looser, "baggier," and more wrinkly. The skin of the scrotal sac takes on a different texture, or "feel." In fair-skinned boys, the skin on the penis and scrotal sac gets rather reddish. Darker-skinned boys, too, will notice that the skin on their genitals gets deeper in color during this stage.

The penis doesn't get much larger during this stage. The most noticeable change in Stage 2 is the size of the testicles and the scrotum. Some boys develop pubic hair during this stage, but many boys do not develop pubic hair until Stage 3 or later.

As we explained, different boys begin puberty at different ages. Most boys start Stage 2 at about eleven or twelve, although some start when they are a year or so younger, and some when they are a year or so older than this.

For some boys, it is very clear when they have reached Stage 2 and started puberty. One day they look at their testicles and think, "Oh, wow, they've really gotten bigger." Other boys, especially those who have been watching their bodies closely, are not so sure. They may think, "It *seems* like they're getting bigger, but maybe I'm just imagining it."

Still other boys get to feeling kind of discouraged because puberty seems to be happening so slowly to them. They're eager to have mature, muscular bodies, and all that's happening is a little bit of growth in their testicles. If you start feeling down in the dumps because your body isn't changing as fast as you'd like, it helps to remember that all those changes you're waiting for *will* eventually happen.

If you're not certain if you've begun Stage 2, you might want to take a look at the orchidometer in Illustration 10. This is an actual, life-size drawing of an orchidometer, a tool doctors invented to study the different stages of puberty. It is a rather specialized tool, though, and not every doctor has one. It is a series of wooden or plastic egg-shaped ovals that are strung together on a cord in order of increasing size, from the smallest to the largest. If you were to hold the orchidometer in one hand and one of your testicles in the other hand, you would be able to see which of the ovals is closest in size to your testicle. Maybe you can get an idea of which you are closest to just by looking at the drawing and feeling one of your testicles.

The number written on each oval of the orchidometer shows the volume of that oval. *Volume* means "how

orchidometer (OR-ki-DOM-e-ter)

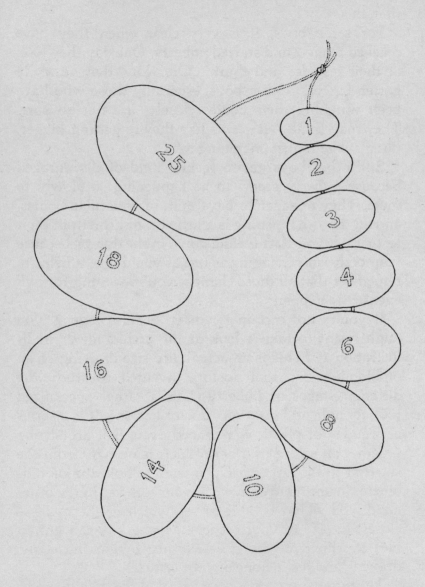

Illustration 10. Orchidometer, actual size

much something can hold," and it is a way of measuring size. The first oval on the orchidometer, the one marked 1, has a volume of one milliliter, which is about one-fifth of a teaspoon. The last oval, the one marked 25, has a volume of twenty-five milliliters, or about five teaspoons.

Fully grown men have testicles between sixteen and twenty-seven milliliters in volume. Boys who have not yet started puberty—that is, boys who are only in Stage 1—have testicles that are about the size of the 1, 2, or 3 ovals. If your testicle is the size of the 4 oval or larger, this means that you have reached Stage 2 and have officially begun puberty.

Stage 3
By the time a boy reaches Stage 3, his penis has begun to get bigger too. As you can tell from Illustration 9, the penis gets quite a bit larger than it was in Stage 1 or 2. It gets both longer and wider. The scrotum and testicles also grow during this stage, but the most noticeable change is in the size of the penis. The skin of the penis and scrotum also continues to deepen in color.

By the time a boy's penis has started to grow larger, his testicles are usually between seven and sixteen milliliters in volume (see the orchidometer in Illustration 10), although some boys in Stage 3 have testicles that are larger or smaller than this.

One testicle usually hangs lower than the other. In most grown men, it is the left testicle that hangs lower, but in some it is the right. If you have not noticed one testicle hanging lower than the other by the time you get to Stage 3, you will probably notice it during this stage.

The reason one testicle hangs lower than the other is to keep them from crushing each other when you walk.

If you have ever been hit in the testicles, you know that they are *very* sensitive. It can be really painful if your testicles get crushed together or if you get hit there. That is why boys often wear jockstraps or cup-shaped protectors in gym class or when they are playing sports (see Illustration 11). The jockstrap or cup holds the testicles snugly up against the body so that they are not hanging out and are protected from injury.

In grown men, both testicles are just about the same size, although sometimes one may be just a bit larger than the other. As you are developing, you may notice that one testicle is a good bit larger than the other. This is because one testicle may grow a bit faster. Often, the one that hangs lower is the largest. As the other grows, it may start to hang lower. So a boy who notices that his right testicle hangs lower in Stage 3 may find that his left testicle hangs lower in Stage 4. (If you are concerned about the difference in the size of your testicles or notice a sudden, dramatic change in size or in which

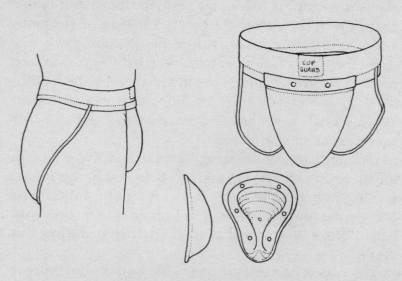

Illustration 11. Cup protector

one is lowest, see the section on testicular self-examination, page 204.)

If a boy has not already started to develop pubic hair in Stage 2, he may notice the first curly hairs growing around the base of his penis during Stage 3. The first pubic hairs are not usually very dark in color or really curly. There aren't very many at first, and you may have to look very closely to see them. But as puberty continues, they will get darker in color and there will be more of them. They begin growing around the base of the penis, just where the penis joins the body. After a while, they start growing on the scrotum as well. They may also grow in the area around the anus.

Some of the boys and men we talked to were a bit worried when they started to grow pubic hair. Here is what some of them had to say:

> It looked like I was getting all these pimples on the skin around my cock.
>
> Jim, age 16

> There were little raised bumps, and I thought I had some kind of disease.
>
> Phil, age 24

> First I got these tiny, kind of whitish, raised spots. I was scared to say anything. I just waited. Then I noticed these fuzzy hairs growing out.
>
> Bill, age 17

When pubic hair starts to grow, there are often raised bumps on the surface of the skin that may look like pimples. These raised bumps are caused by the tiny pubic hairs trying to push through the skin. Soon, little hairs begin to poke through the surface of the bumps. If you don't know what is going on, it can be a bit scary. But it is a perfectly normal part of growing up, and it is not anything to worry about.

You may also notice that you have other little bumps or dots on the skin of the penis and scrotum, ones that do not grow little hairs. These are oil and perspiration (sweat) glands. They begin to develop during puberty and to make small amounts of oil and perspiration. You may notice that the skin in this area feels moister or smells a bit different. This is because your oil and sweat glands are becoming active. Once again, this is a normal and natural part of growing up, another sign that you are becoming a man.

Just as it is impossible to say when a boy will reach Stage 2 and start puberty, so it is impossible to say when he will reach Stage 3. The usual age is about thirteen, although there are some who reach Stage 3 when they are younger than this, and some who reach it when they are older.

Stage 4

As you can see from Illustration 9 (page 29), by the time a boy reaches Stage 4, his penis has gotten quite a bit larger. It is both wider and longer, and the glans, or head, of the penis is more developed. The scrotum hangs lower and the testicles are also larger. The testicles are usually about 1½ inches long by the time a boy has reached this stage, and they are usually between twelve and twenty-four milliliters in volume (see Illustration 9)—although some boys' testicles will be slightly smaller or larger than this in Stage 4.

During this stage, the skin of the scrotal sac and penis continues to get deeper in color. The oil and sweat glands continue to develop too. The usual age at which boys reach Stage 4 is about fourteen, although again some boys will be younger than this and some will be older.

Most boys will have quite a bit of pubic hair by the

time they reach Stage 4. As a boy continues to develop, the pubic hair gets curlier, coarser, and darker in color. It usually grows in an upside-down triangle pattern on the lower part of his belly, around the base of the penis. In many boys, the pubic hair continues to grow up toward the belly button and out toward the thighs. As we mentioned before, it may also grow on the scrotum and around the anus.

Your pubic hair is often the same color as the hair on your head, but it may also be a lighter or darker color. When you become an old man, the pubic hair, like the hair on your head, is apt to turn gray.

Stage 5

This is the adult or fully grown stage. The testicles are usually about 1¾ inches long. They are generally between sixteen and twenty-seven milliliters in volume (see Illustration 10). The scrotal sac is also fully developed by the time a boy reaches this stage. And the skin of the scrotum and penis has gotten even deeper in color.

A grown man's penis is usually between 3¼ and 4¼ inches in length. When a man or boy has an erection, his penis gets temporarily larger. The largest erect penis ever recorded by a doctor was 12 inches long. The smallest was 4¾ inches. Ninety out of 100 men will have a penis that is between 5 and 7 inches in length when it is erect, with the average length being about 6¼ inches. The smaller a penis is when it is soft, the more inches it tends to gain when it becomes erect. For example, a man with a penis that measures 3 inches when it is soft may add as many as 3¼ inches when his penis becomes hard. A man with a penis that measures 4¼ inches when soft might add only 2 inches during an erection. Thus, even though the lengths of their penises were different when they were soft, both men would have a 6¼-inch penis when they had erections. (We will talk more about penis size in Chapter 3.)

The penis may also get temporarily smaller from time to time. You may have noticed that your penis gets a little smaller if you jump into a cold bath or shower. Cold weather, being really tired out, or feeling nervous may also make your penis shrivel up a bit. Any of these things may also make your scrotal sac pull up closer to your body and seem temporarily smaller. In old age, the penis tends to become a bit smaller in size permanently.

The average age that boys reach Stage 5 is about sixteen, although as with Stages 2 through 4, there will be boys who enter Stage 5 when they are younger, and some when they are older.

The pubic hair is also fairly well developed by Stage 5. But pubic hair may continue to grow until the boy reaches the age of twenty.

Some boys have quite a bit of pubic hair; others have very little. How much you have will probably depend on your family. If the men in your family have lots of hair, you probably will too. If the men in your family are not especially hairy, chances are you will not be either. Again, this is not a hard and fast rule, but boys often take after their fathers in this way.

HOW LONG DOES IT TAKE TO GET THROUGH THESE STAGES?

There is no simple answer to this question because each boy is different. But doctors have studied boys going through puberty, so we can tell you about what happens to *most* boys.

As you may recall from the beginning of this chapter,

the earlier starters do not necessarily go through these stages any faster than boys who start puberty later or boys who start at the average age. Boys may take anywhere from a year to six years to go from Stage 2, the beginning of puberty, to Stage 5, the fully grown adult stage. The so-called average boy takes about four years. The table you see below shows how long boys take to go through each of the various stages of genital development. The first column shows how long the *average* boy takes to go through each stage. But, as we've said, not all boys are average. The second column shows the range of times it takes *most* boys to go through these stages.

THE LENGTH OF TIME BOYS SPEND IN STAGES 2, 3, AND 4

	The "Average" Boy	The Range of Times for 97 Out of 100 Boys
Stage 2	About 13 months	About 5 months to about 26 months
Stage 3	About 10 months	About 2 months to about 19 months
Stage 4	About 24 months	About 5 months to about 36 months

Let's say you are twelve years old and have just reached Stage 2. If you are a so-called typical or average boy, you will probably reach Stage 3 in about thirteen more months; that is, in one year and one month. However, you may be quick to develop and may find yourself in Stage 3 in only five months. Or you may be slower to develop and may not find yourself in Stage 3 until twenty-six months (two years and two months) have gone by. This table will not tell you exactly when the various changes that happen during puberty are going to happen to you, but it will give you some idea of what to expect.

FEELINGS ABOUT STARTING PUBERTY

Boys (and girls too) have all sorts of feelings about starting puberty. I've noticed that the kids in my youngest class (third and fourth graders), who haven't started puberty yet, are often excited about and looking forward to the changes that will take place in their bodies. But not everyone feels this way. As one third grader put it:

> Ugh! I don't want my penis to get all big and hairy and ugly looking!

By and large, though, the younger kids are really eager to grow up. They're curious about the changes that will take place and generally feel comfortable about asking questions in class. They don't use the Everything You Ever Wanted to Know question box as often as the older kids do. They just ask their questions right out loud.

The older kids who are about to start or have just started puberty are usually excited too. They often feel very proud when they notice their bodies starting to change. As one boy said:

> It's a "Hey, whoopee, I'm finally growing up!" kind of feeling.

But I've noticed that the older kids don't feel quite as comfortable about asking questions right out loud. As a group, they seem to feel more embarrassed about puberty than the younger kids. Even the kids who were in my class in third or fourth grade, and who were especially open and comfortable talking about the body changes of puberty, often seem more modest and rather shy about things by the time they're in sixth or seventh grade.

I think this difference I've noticed between the younger kids and the older ones is due, at least in part, to the fact that by the time you get to sixth or seventh grade, puberty is no longer some far-off thing that's going to happen someday. It's actually happening to *you*, and it's happening right now. It's much more personal, and this can make it harder to talk about.

I think, too, that once the changes have actually started to happen, most of us have some doubtful or uncertain feelings mixed in with our excited, proud feelings. Having mixed feelings about going through puberty is quite normal. Almost everyone has some doubts. One boy said it particularly well:

I was taking a bath with my sister and she said, "What's that?" and I saw that I had some pubic hairs. I guess my penis and balls had been getting bigger all along. It wasn't till my sister saw the pubic hair that I really realized I was changing. I felt grown up and I was really jazzed about it. Then, two seconds later, I had this really scared feeling . . . "Oh, no, I'm not ready for this."

Many of the men and boys we interviewed remembered having these "I'm-not-ready" feelings. If you have these feelings, it helps to remember that it's quite normal to have them. In Chapter 9, we talk more about the kinds of feelings people have about going through puberty.

Some of the boys and men we talked to who started puberty late said that this had affected them. As one man explained:

I didn't go through puberty until I was sixteen. It really bothered me when I was in situations where other boys could see that I hadn't started yet. I was always embarrassed in gym class and I always tried to hide my body.

Jim, age 47

Another man told us:

I was a late starter, too. It seemed like all the other guys had really developed bodies and hair all over the place, and here I was still a skinny, little kid. Once it started, though, I really developed fast. My whole attitude was, "Thank God! At last it's happening to me." For a while there, I was thinking it would never happen and that maybe I was some kind of freak or maybe I was sick or there was something wrong. But, finally, I started to develop, too.

Glenn, age 42

Sometimes the boys and men who started earlier than the other guys had embarrassed feelings, too:

I developed at a very early age. I was really proud, but also embarrassed because I looked so different from the other kids. It's hard at that age to be different. You want to be just like the other guys and not stand out.

Pete, age 26

Even boys who started at the usual age sometimes felt embarrassed or uncertain about the changes taking place in their bodies, especially if they hadn't been told what to expect. Everyone we talked to, whether they felt proud and excited or uncertain and embarrassed (or a bit of both), agreed that it helps to have some idea of what to expect and to have someone to talk to about your feelings. Reading this book with someone might be a good way to start talking about these things.

AM I NORMAL?

As we're going through puberty, we may worry about whether everything is going according to plan. Sometimes puberty seems to be going very slowly. The changes in our bodies may be so slight as we move from stage to stage, especially in the early stages, that we wonder if we're really growing at all. We may ask ourselves, "Am I normal?" If you've started puberty, but your growth isn't as fast or dramatic as you'd like, hang in there. You *will* continue to grow and eventually you will have a fully mature adult body.

Boys who are late starters may also ask themselves, "Am I normal?" If they don't start puberty until two or three years after most of their friends have started, they often worry that maybe there's something wrong with them, that they have some kind of medical problem. But being a late starter doesn't usually mean there's anything physically wrong with you. It just means that your body is developing at a slower rate than most other boys' bodies.

Every once in a while, though, there are boys who are late starters not because they are simply slow to develop but because there is actually something physically wrong with them. Such boys need to see a doctor. Doctors have ways of treating these problems so that the boy will go through the normal body changes of puberty.

You may be wondering how you'd know if you were just a late starter or if you had a medical problem that needs a doctor's attention. We tell boys that if they've reached the age of fifteen and haven't started to go through any of the puberty changes described in this chapter, they should see a doctor. For example, a boy who was still in Stage 1 of genital development (see Illustration 9 on page 29) and who didn't have any pubic hair by age fifteen should see a doctor. Now, it doesn't necessarily mean that you have a medical problem if you haven't started to go through any of the body changes of puberty by the age of fifteen. There are some perfectly healthy boys who don't go through puberty until their late teens. But not starting by fifteen *may* mean you have a problem that needs medical attention, so it's a good idea to get it checked out.

By the way, if you have a feeling that something isn't right with the way your body is developing, you don't *have* to wait until you're fifteen to see a doctor. If you go to see a doctor before fifteen and it turns out that you do have a problem, you'll have caught the problem that much earlier. If you don't have a problem, you'll feel better knowing that you're just a late starter and that there's nothing wrong with you.

It's not just late starters who worry; boys who are early do too. But in most cases, being an early starter doesn't mean there's anything wrong with you. It just means that your body is developing a bit faster than other boys' bodies. However, just as being a late starter is occasionally a sign of a medical problem, so being an especially early starter can be a sign that something's wrong. If you begin puberty before the age of nine, it's a good idea to see a doctor to make sure that you don't have a problem.

KEEPING TRACK OF YOUR PROGRESS

Some of the boys in my classes get really interested in the stages of puberty. They study the five stages shown in Illustration 9 and compare their testicles to the orchidometer in Illustration 10. They pore over the

MY PUBERTY CHART

Date: _____
Height: _____ Weight: _____
Stage of Genital
Development: _____
Pubic Hair: _____
Facial Hair: _____
Other Changes: _____

_____
_____
_____
_____

Date: _____
Height: _____ Weight: _____
Stage of Genital
Development: _____
Pubic Hair: _____
Facial Hair: _____
Other Changes: _____

_____
_____
_____
_____

Date: _____
Height: _____ Weight: _____
Stage of Genital
Development: _____
Pubic Hair: _____
Facial Hair: _____
Other Changes: _____

_____
_____
_____
_____

Date: _____
Height: _____ Weight: _____
Stage of Genital
Development: _____
Pubic Hair: _____
Facial Hair: _____
Other Changes: _____

_____
_____
_____
_____

Date: _____
Height: _____ Weight: _____
Stage of Genital
Development: _____
Pubic Hair: _____
Facial Hair: _____
Other Changes: _____

_____
_____
_____
_____

Date: _____
Height: _____ Weight: _____
Stage of Genital
Development: _____
Pubic Hair: _____
Facial Hair: _____
Other Changes: _____

_____
_____
_____
_____

table on page 39 and try to figure out what stage they're at and when to expect other changes. Some of the boys in my class, however, couldn't care less. They figure that these changes are going to happen whether or not they pay attention to them, so why should they bother trying to follow it. You may be like the curious boys in my class, or you may be like those who are not as interested. If you *are* the type who likes to keep track of things, you might want to keep a record of your progress through puberty by using the chart on page 45. Before you fill out the chart, though, you might want to read the next few chapters, which talk about some of the other changes that happen to a boy's body during puberty.

How to Use the Puberty Chart

Start by filling in the first section of the chart. Write the date and record your height and weight. Then, turn back to Illustration 9 on page 29 and decide which stage of genital development you're closest to at the moment. Write the number of that stage on the appropriate line. On the Pubic Hair line, write "none" if you don't have any pubic hair yet. Or, if you have pubic hair already, write "a few hairs," "some dark, curly hairs," "lots of hair," or some other descriptive words. On the Facial Hair line, write "none" if you don't have any. If you've begun to develop a few dark hairs on the corner of your lip, your cheeks, or some other place, make a note on this line of the chart.

Some of the other puberty changes you might write about in the Other Changes section of the chart are:

body odor

more erections

greater strength

hairier arms and legs

broader shoulders

amount of perspiration

pimples

breast swelling or tenderness

stronger sexual feelings

more muscles

oilier hair and skin

voice changes

ejaculation

Every three months or so, or every time you notice a big change, fill in a new section of the chart.

Keeping track of the changes that happen during puberty can give you more of a sense of being on top of things. It might be fun to do the chart with your mom or dad, with a friend, or with someone else close to you. Since fathers and sons are often alike in the way they go through puberty, you may want to keep this book and the charts you have filled in and pass them along to your own son if you have one someday.

CHAPTER 3

Changing Size and Shape

People often say that girls start puberty a year or two before boys, and I must admit that I used to think the same thing. I was really surprised to learn that the first puberty changes that take place in girls (the development of their sex organs, the growth of pubic hair, and the development of their breasts) happen at just about the same age that the first puberty changes in boys (the changes in the testicles, and the growth of pubic hair) begin to take place.

People get the idea that girls start puberty earlier than boys for two reasons. First of all, when a girl's breasts start to develop, we can see that this change is happening even though she is fully clothed. Most boys' testicles are starting to grow at the same time, but unless we see a boy naked, we are not aware of this change in his body in the way we are aware of a girl's breast development. Besides, the change in a boy's testicles is just not as dramatic as the changes that take place in a girl's body at the very beginning of puberty.

The second reason people think that girls go through puberty earlier than boys has to do with the "puberty growth spurt." During puberty, both boys and girls begin to grow taller at a faster rate, and a girl's growth spurt usually happens about two years before a boy's. This gives people the idea that girls start puberty before boys. But the growth spurt is just one of the changes that happen during puberty. The other puberty changes—things like the development of sex organs, of pubic hair, and, in girls, of the breasts—happen at about the same age in both boys and girls. Of course, some boys and girls are early starters and some are late starters, so everyone doesn't start at the same time. Still, the average boy and the average girl begin puberty at just about the same age.

THE GROWTH SPURT— WHEN AND HOW MUCH?

In girls, the growth spurt is sometimes the first change that happens during puberty. In boys, however, it rarely happens until the sex organs have begun to develop. Most boys start to notice the growth spurt between the ages of thirteen and fourteen, although some boys are somewhat younger or older when it starts.

Beginning at about the age of two, most children grow about two inches taller each year until they reach puberty. When the growth spurt begins, it may be very dramatic. Some boys add as many as five inches a year to their height during the growth spurt. Or the growth spurt may not be so sudden and noticeable. Some boys grow only about 2½ inches a year during the growth spurt. Most boys, though, grow about 3½ inches a year. The growth spurt may last for a few years. Then the rate of growth slows down again. This does not mean that a boy will stop growing altogether; most boys continue to grow taller until they get to about the age of twenty. But the period of extra-fast growth lasts only about three years.

HOW TALL WILL I BE?

A lot of boys want to know if there is any way that they can tell exactly how tall they will be when they are grown-up. Unfortunately, there isn't, but there are some clues that may help you make a rough guess. How tall you are usually has to do with your family. If both your parents are tall, chances are you will be too. If both your parents are short, you will probably be short. This is not a hard and fast rule, though—there are lots and lots of exceptions.

The tallest man who ever lived was eight feet, eleven inches tall, and the shortest was only 26½ inches. But these were unusual cases; 95 out of 100 men will be between five feet, four inches and six feet, two inches tall. The average height for grown men is five feet, nine inches tall.

By the way, don't make the mistake of thinking that boys who are on the short side before puberty will be shorter than the other men when they reach their adult heights. It is true that many boys who are short before puberty are short as adults, but this is not always the case. As one man said:

In eighth grade, I was the second-to-the-shortest kid in the class, but over the summer, I shot up. By the time I started ninth grade, I was just about the tallest boy in the class.

John, age 26

No one can say for sure which boys will end up being taller than average and which ones will end up being shorter than average—or, for that matter, which ones will end up being just about average. But we do know that by the age of ten, the average boy will have grown to 78 percent of his adult height and that by age fourteen, the average boy will have grown to 91.5 percent of his adult height. (*Percent* means "part of a hundred." A boy who reached his full height would have reached 100 percent of his adult height. A boy who had reached half his full height would have reached 50 percent of his adult height.)

CHANGING SHAPE

Illustration 12 shows an adult man and a baby boy. As you can see, we do quite a bit of growing between the time we're born and the time we reach our full adult size. For one thing, we get taller. As explained before, a lot of this growing taller happens during puberty. We also put on quite a bit of weight. At birth, the average boy baby weighs 7½ pounds. The average grown man weighs 162 pounds. Again, a lot of this weight gain happens during puberty.

If you compare the baby's body to the man's body, you'll see that some parts of the body grow more than others as we mature and grow into our adult bodies. If this weren't true, if all parts of our bodies grew the same amount as we matured, we'd simply grow into giant babies, and we'd look pretty strange. If you take a look at Illustration 13, you'll see what I mean.

Of course, we don't end up looking like giant babies. Different parts of our bodies grow more or less than other parts in proportion (in comparison to) other parts. For example, our heads don't grow as much as

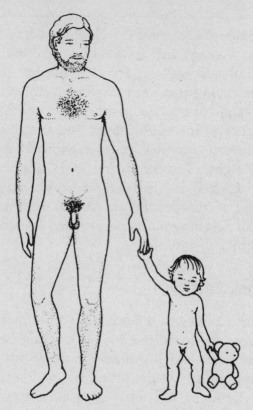

Illustration 12. Adult male and infant male

other parts of our body. During puberty, you may notice changes in the proportions or the size of certain parts of your body in relation to other parts. For instance, the proportions of your face change. The lower part gets longer, and this changes the general shape of your face.

Your shoulders also get broader, and your hips seem narrower in comparison to your broad shoulders. Your shoulders become more muscular. In fact, the muscles all over your body grow larger, especially in your thighs, calves, and upper arms. With this increase in the size of your muscles comes an increase in body

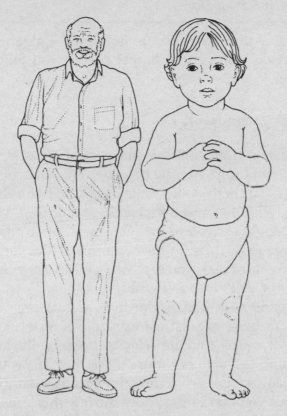

Illustration 13. Adult male and giant baby

strength. Your whole body begins to look less like a boy's body and more like a man's. Your arms and legs tend to grow faster than your backbone during your growth spurt. So you may notice that your arms and legs are longer in proportion to the trunk of your body than they were during childhood or than they are in adulthood. The bones in your feet also grow faster than your other bones, and so your feet usually reach their adult size before you reach your full height. Some boys whose feet are already quite large but who are still going through the growth spurt think that their feet are going to continue to grow as they get taller.

They worry that their feet are going to be gigantic. But your feet do stop getting bigger before you finish getting taller.

LIKING YOUR BODY

Bodies come in all sorts of shapes and sizes—short or tall, thin or plump, narrow or wide, muscular or not so muscular. To some extent, you can change the shape of your body by diet and exercise. If you're thin, you can put on weight. If you're fat, you can diet so that your body loses some if its fat tissue. If you'd like your body to be more muscular, you can lift weights or work out in a gym once you've started puberty. Doing slow, repetitious exercises, in which you lift weights or use your muscles to push against a heavy piece of gym equipment, will cause your muscles to become thicker and shorter and to bulge out more. (You have to wait until you've started puberty, though, because without the hormones your body produces during this time—we'll talk more about these in Chapter 4—your muscles won't respond to the exercise.) But remember that you do have a basic body shape that can't be changed no matter how much or how little you eat or what type of exercise you do.

If you aren't satisfied with your body and are under- or overweight, perhaps you need to see a doctor and get on a diet and exercise plan to help you gain or lose weight. If you are not sure whether you're under- or overweight, your doctor can help you decide if your weight is within the normal ranges for age, height, and body build. If you fall within the normal ranges and still aren't satisfied with the way your body looks, maybe you need to think about where you've gotten these ideas about how your body *should* look, ideas that are making you feel dissatisfied with the way you *do* look.

It would be nice if we could all just look at our bodies without having to compare them to someone else's and say, "Hey, I like the way I look." But we live in a society where there's a lot of competition among people, companies, and even countries. We're always comparing and competing to see who's best. So who decides what's best?

Most of us get our ideas about what's the "best" or "most attractive" kind of male body from the pictures we see in magazines, on billboards, and in television and the movies. Right now in our country, these pictures often show tall men with big, bulging muscles, handsome, regular features, no pimples, slim waists, small rear ends, and hairy chests. As you may have noticed, not too many men actually look like this.

When we are constantly bombarded with pictures of these tall, muscular, handsome men, we can get the feeling that there's something about our bodies that is somehow not right. If we don't look like them, we may be unhappy with the way we look. After all, if these are the men who are always the heros in the movies, always getting the girls or winding up being successful, what message does that send to those of us who aren't tall, muscular, or good-looking in that particular way? With all these images of perfect "hunks," it's easy to get to thinking that their bodies actually *are* better or more attractive. If you feel this way sometimes, it helps to remember that these bodies seem more desirable only because they are in fashion in our particular culture at this particular time. Being in fashion doesn't make a miniskirt "better" than a knee-length skirt, and being in fashion doesn't make one body type better than another.

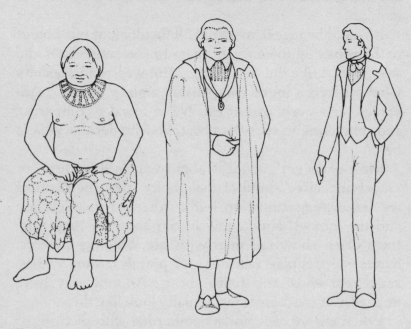

Illustration 14. Fashions in appearance. From the left are a Polynesian king, a seventeenth-century German burghermeister, and a nineteenth-century Englishman.

It helps, too, to remember that fashions change and that they vary from culture to culture. Illustration 14 shows bodies that have been in fashion in other times and other cultures. The first drawing is a Polynesian king. Most people in our society would find him grossly overweight, yet in his culture he's considered a fine figure of a man. His huge belly is taken as a sign of his masculinity. The seventeenth-century German burghermeister in the second picture would also be considered a bit chunky by our standards, yet in his own day and age his bulk was considered attractive, a sign of his success and prosperity. The third fellow is an Englishman from the nineteenth century. His thin, narrow body and lack of muscles make him look rather fragile in comparison to the hunk kind of body now in fashion in our country. Yet back then, in England, he was the type of guy who had women swooning over him. In fact, back then, one of our modern-day hunks might have been considered a real barbarian and not at all attractive.

It also helps to remember that not everyone agrees with or goes along with the fashions of the day. For instance, there are plenty of women who find men with huge muscles popping out all over grossly unattractive. Many women prefer thin men. And for most people, it's not what kind of body you have but what kind of person you are that really counts.

Learning to appreciate yourself and to like your own body, regardless of whether or not it matches up to what's in fashion, is a big step in growing up. If you find your own body attractive, other people will too.

Of course, it isn't always easy to learn to like your own body. Even though most of the boys we talked to were pleased about the fact that their bodies were changing and becoming adult, they sometimes wished that they were taller or wider across the chest, or more muscular, or more something else. We asked the men we interviewed, "Have you ever wished your body were different in some way, and if so, how?", or "What's the one thing you would most like to change about your body?" We got many different answers, but two topics came up more than the others, so we'd like to talk a bit about them.

Height
One thing that men mentioned over and over again was their height. Except for those who were very tall, almost all of the men we interviewed said they wished they

were a bit taller. Even if they were average height (five feet, nine inches) or a couple of inches taller than average, they often said they "wouldn't mind" being a bit taller. The men who were shorter than average almost always said they wished they were taller. As one man put it:

I'm only five feet, six inches, and being short has always bugged me. People make cracks, call you "shrimp" or "shortie." I'm really coordinated and good at sports. Being short made it difficult to get on the team in high school. I guess I compensated by getting into weight lifting and concentrating on wrestling. In a way, though, now that I'm older, it turns out that being short was kind of an advantage because it made really concentrating on working out and developing a strong, muscular body a habit that's stayed with me. I still work out and I'm in great physical shape, whereas a lot of guys my age, the ones who were tall in high school and all, are overweight and flabby and out of shape. I'm healthier than a lot of guys, and maybe if I'd been taller I wouldn't have gotten so into working out and taking care of my body. Still, to tell the truth, I wish I were taller.

Harold, age 34

Another man had this to say:

No doubt about it, being tall is an advantage. People look up to you. I think being short is a disadvantage, in sports, with girls . . . and in other ways. Short guys have a lot of problems to contend with that just aren't there for tall guys.

Hank, age 20

Not all short men are bothered by their lack of height:

I've always been short, even as a kid, so I've had a whole lifetime to adjust, and it's really not a problem for me like it is for some guys. I know lots of short guys who are always kind of cocky, on the defensive, who talk loud or always act the clown or are kind of brash or pushy. They're sort of making up for the fact that they're short, acting big so that people will notice them, like they might get missed or passed over because they're short. But I don't really feel that need. I'm short and I'm a pretty quiet guy, but I still feel that people take note of me because I'm comfortable with myself the way I am. I think people notice or feel that kind of satisfaction when you're at peace with yourself and accept yourself the way you are.

Rick, age 39

And tall men aren't always happy about their height:

I'm six foot seven, and I'm always looking down on other people. People are always saying dumb things like, "How is the weather up there?" I was this tall when I was fourteen, and I always felt like a freak. I kind of slouched and hunched over, trying not to look so tall. My mother was always yelling at me to stand up straight. I still have terrible posture. I'm in my forties now, so it's not so bad anymore. There are little inconveniences, like bumping your head and trying to scrunch into cars, but it's not like when I was a teenager. It really bothered me then. Being different was difficult.

Frank, age 43

But being short can pose problems, as Rick explains:

There's a sort of unwritten rule that the guy has to be taller than the girl. All the girls were always taller than me, so I realized early on that I wasn't going to pay attention to that rule because if I only asked out girls who were shorter than me . . . well, I wouldn't have gone out on too many dates. So I just ignored that rule and asked out whomever I wanted. I got turned down sometimes, just on account of my height. There were girls, and later women, who even though they'd go out with me were bothered by my being short. They'd wear flat-heeled shoes instead of the high heels they probably would have worn. But once I got involved with someone, you know, seriously, we'd kid around and it was never a real problem. It's true that a lot of people follow this rule about the guy having to be taller, and it does affect you. Maybe it's a little harder to get a date, to find a girl who isn't uptight about it. My wife, by the way, is five inches taller than me and wears high heels, and it doesn't bother her that there's a difference in our height. It is breaking that unwritten law, though, and people do look at us. I figure that's their problem.

Rick, age 39

Rick has a healthy attitude about himself and doesn't seem to worry about what other people think. But there's no getting around the fact that our society attaches a lot of importance to a man's height. In fact, many people are prejudiced against short men. You're probably familiar with racial prejudice. People who have racial prejudices make judgments about or discriminate against people whose skin is a different color from theirs. They prejudge (*prejudice* means "to prejudge") people of other races and make assumptions about what they are like before they even meet or get to know anything about them as individuals. Prejudice against short men isn't as obvious or as talked about as racial prejudice, but it does exist and can cause problems. For example, studies have shown that if two equally qualified men apply for a job and one is tall and the other short, the tall man is more likely to get the job, simply because he's tall.

In other studies, researchers have given people pictures of a tall man and a short man and asked them to write descriptions of what they think these men are like based on the pictures. The researchers found that people tend to describe the tall man in more positive terms, using words like "brave," "sincere," "handsome," "successful," and so on. They tend to describe the short man in less positive or even negative terms: "not so successful," "insecure," "dishonest," and so forth.

Given the kinds of prejudices some (not all, but some) people have, it's not surprising that short men often wish they were taller. The truth of the matter is that your height doesn't have anything to do with your worth as a person, and it doesn't have anything to do with how successful you may become. Think of the many shorter-than-average men who have become famous stars, men like actors Dustin Hoffman and Dudley Moore, and baseball greats Phil Rizzuto and Joe Morgan, among many others. Of course, knowing this fact intellectually is a lot easier than really believing it with your heart and feeling okay about yourself if you're short. It helps to remember what Rick said about people responding to a person who has the inner satisfaction and confidence that comes from accepting himself the way he is. It's true. If you learn to accept yourself, to take pride in your unique self, then other people will too.

Penis Size

The other thing that often came up when we asked men how they felt about their bodies was the issue of penis size. Perhaps you've heard people make jokes about this subject. Or maybe you have been in the showers in the gym locker room and heard boys teasing other boys about the size of their penis. Maybe you have done this kind of teasing yourself, or you have been teased in this way.

If any of these things have happened to you, you're not alone. However, you may never have heard these sorts of jokes or teasing, or wished your penis were larger. If this is the case, you may be wondering what all the fuss is about.

People often make a big deal out of penis size because they believe the many myths that they hear about it. Myths are stories that people believe are true, but, as we shall see, many myths are completely false. Here are some of the myths that people tell about penis size, along with the real facts.

Myth: Tall men with big, husky builds and lots of muscles have bigger penises than short or skinny men.

Fact: The size of your penis doesn't have anything to do with how tall you are, how muscular you are, how much you weigh, or how your body is built. A short skinny man may have a big penis or a small one. A tall husky football player may have a big one or a small one.

Myth: Men with big thumbs have big penises. This myth has many variations: men with big noses, big ears, big feet . . . men with big whatevers.

Fact: The size of your penis has nothing to do with the size of any other part of your body. No one can tell what size your penis is by looking at the size of your thumb, your nose, your feet, your ears, or any other part of your body.

Myth: Men who come from a certain racial or ethnic background have bigger penises. Sometimes this myth specifies a certain race or ethnic group. For example, you may have heard that black men or Italian men have bigger penises.

Fact: There is no scientific evidence to show that men belonging to any one racial or ethnic group have larger penises than men from other races or ethnic groups.

Myth: A man whose penis is shorter than usual when soft has a shorter-than-average penis when erect.

Fact: The size of your penis when it is soft does not really have much to do with the size it is when it is erect. As we explained in Chapter 2, most grown men's penises are about 3¼ to 4¼ inches long when they are soft. Those that are on the short size when they are soft, say 3¼ inches or so, may add about three inches when they are erect. Men whose penises are on the long side, say 4¼ inches, may get only about two inches more during an erection. However, almost everyone, regardless of the size of their penis when soft, adds at least two inches when they are having an erection. So a man whose penis is unusually large when it is soft, say seven inches, might have a nine-inch penis when it is hard. Most men's penises are about 6¼ inches long when they are having an erection, regardless of how long they are when they are soft.

Myth: Men with big penises are more masculine, or "manly," or macho than men with smaller penises. This myth has many variations, depending on what people consider manly or masculine. You may have heard that men who have large penises are better at sports, or braver, or stronger.

Fact: The size of your penis does not have anything to do with how brave or strong or masculine or manly you are.

Myth: Men with big penises make more sperm in their bodies and can get a woman pregnant more easily than men with smaller penises.

Fact: The size of your penis or, for that matter, your testicles has nothing to do with how many sperm your testicles make. If a man with a big penis has sexual intercourse with a woman, she is not any more or less likely to get pregnant than if she had had sex with a man with a small penis.

Myth: If your penis is small, it won't "fit" into a woman's vagina when you are having sexual intercourse. You may also have heard the opposite of this myth: that if a man's penis is too big, it won't fit into the woman's vagina.

Fact: There are certain very rare medical conditions that can cause a man's penis to be abnormally small or abnormally large. But other than these one-in-a-million cases, penises are never too large or too small for a man to have intercourse with a woman. A woman's vagina is only about three to five inches long, but it is very expandable. Recall from Chapter 1 that the vagina can expand enough to allow a baby to pass through it when she is giving birth. Babies weigh anywhere from about five to ten pounds when they are born, so they are considerably larger than any man's penis. It is just not true that a man's penis can be too large.

A woman's vagina is like a balloon with no air in it. The sides rest up against each other, just as the sides of a collapsed balloon do. So even if a man had a very small penis, it would still fit snugly inside a woman's vagina.

Myth: Men with big penises are more sexually powerful. This myth also has many variations: men with big penises have a stronger sexual drive, have a larger sexual appetite, have more erections, or have erections that last longer.

Fact: The size of your penis does not have anything to do with any of these things. Different men have different sexual drives, and some have erections more often than others, but these differences have nothing to do with their penis size.

Myth: Women enjoy sex more if the man has a big penis.

Fact: Penis size has very little to do with how much a woman enjoys sexual intercourse. Women's pleasure in intercourse comes mostly from the stimulation they get in the area around the clitoris and the vaginal opening, rather than inside the vagina. It's also affected by their emotional feelings about their partners. So the size of the penis is of little importance.

With all these myths going around, it's not surprising that men often worry about whether their penis is "big enough" or wish that it were larger. If you've worried about this, it helps to remember that all of these myths are simply that—myths. *They just aren't true.* The size of your penis doesn't have anything to do with how much of a man you are or what kind of a person you are.

We hope that the information we've given you so far will help you feel easier about the changes taking place in your body. We hope it will help you learn to accept and like your body, regardless of whether you're tall or short, have a big penis or a small one, are muscular or aren't so muscular. Remember, it's the person inside the body, not the body itself, that's important. If you learn to feel good about your body, other people will too.

CHAPTER 4

Body Hair, Whiskers, Beards, Mustaches, Perspiration, Pimples, and Other Puberty Changes

If the increase in the size of your penis and testicles and the growth spurt were the only things that happened during puberty, Dane and I could have ended this book right here. But, as you may have guessed, there are also other changes that go on in your body during puberty. In this chapter and the next, we will be talking about some of these other changes.

THE ROLE OF HORMONES

You may be wondering what causes all these changes. The fact of the matter is that no one knows for sure, but we do know that it has something to do with *hormones*. Hormones are substances that are made by parts of our bodies called glands. The hormones made in our various glands travel to other parts of our bodies and tell those parts how to develop and grow, or how to work and behave properly.

Our bodies have a number of different glands making dozens of different hormones, most of which have long, tongue-twisting names that you can hardly pronounce, let alone spell. You could go crazy trying to remember the names of all these glands and hormones. But we don't want you to go crazy, so we're only going to talk about the glands and hormones that have the most to do with puberty.

Puberty starts in your brain. A few years before your sex organs start to grow larger or you start to go through your growth spurt, glands in your brain start making larger and larger amounts of certain hormones. One of these glands in your brain is called the *pituitary gland*. The pituitary makes a hormone that gets into your bloodstream and travels to your testicles. As you get older, your pituitary sends more and more of its hormones to your testicles. Your testicles are also glands. The hormones from your brain cause your testicles to make hormones of their own. The most important hormone your testicles make is *testosterone*.

As you begin to go through puberty, your testicles (in response to greater amounts of brain hormones) make increasing amounts of testosterone. The testosterone travels to other parts of your body and tells those parts how to grow and develop. For instance, it is testosterone that causes your penis, testicles, and scrotum to

hormones (HOR-moans)
pituitary (pih-TOO-eh-tear-ee)
testosterone (tes-TOS-tur-own)

grow larger. Testosterone is also responsible for the growth of those curly, crisp pubic hairs. In fact, testosterone plays a role in almost all of the changes we will be talking about in this chapter and the next.

BODY HAIR

In addition to those curly pubic hairs, testosterone also causes hair to grow on other parts of your body. As you're going through puberty, you may notice that you have more hair on your arms, your thighs, and your lower legs. This hair probably won't be as curly as your pubic hair. But there will usually be more hair in these areas of your body than there was during childhood. Hair may also start to grow on your chest. Some boys grow hair on their shoulders and/or their backs. Some grow hair on the backs of their hands. Some boys become really hairy; others have very little body hair.

People often think that the amount of body hair a man has is related to how much testosterone his testicles make. This isn't true. Testosterone causes your body hair to *start* to grow, but how much or how little a man has doesn't have anything to do with how much testosterone his body makes. The amount of body hair you'll have is determined by two things: your racial or ethnic group and your family. As a group, Caucasian (white) men generally have more body hair than Oriental or Negro (black) men. Within any of these groups, the amount of hair a man has usually depends on his family. Boys who come from families in which the men tend to have lots of hair usually wind up having a lot of body hair. Boys who come from families in which the men have little or no hair on their chests, arms, legs, hands, and so forth usually have very little hair. Once again, this isn't a hard and fast rule, but hairiness (or lack of hair) does tend to, as they say, "run in families."

Just as there are a lot of myths about penis size, so there are a lot of myths about body hair. Some people believe that men who have a lot of body hair are more manly or masculine than men who don't have so much. This is nonsense. Body hair (or lack of body hair) doesn't have anything to do with how much of a man you are. Some people (both men *and* women) find lots of body hair attractive. For them, body hair is especially sexy. Others feel that smoother, more hairless bodies are more attractive. But for most people, it doesn't matter that much one way or the other. So if you've worried about the amount of body hair you have, you probably shouldn't bother. For one thing, worrying won't make any difference. Besides, anyone who is going to decide whether or not they like you on the basis of how much body hair you have probably isn't worth knowing anyhow.

FACIAL HAIR

As a boy goes through puberty, he also starts to grow hair on his face. His mustache, sideburns, whiskers, and beard begin to develop. The first of this facial hair doesn't usually appear until a boy's sex organs are fairly well-developed, usually during Stage 4 of genital development (see Illustration 9 on page 29). The average boy will develop his first facial hair between the ages of fourteen and sixteen. A few boys, though, will notice this hair before they're thirteen, and some don't get any until they're nineteen or twenty.

Usually, the first facial hairs will appear at the outer corners of your upper lip. In the beginning, they may be only slightly dark in color and there will only be a few of them. As you get older, they will get deeper in color and there will be more of them. Your mustache will gradually fill out, growing from the outer corners toward the middle of your lips. At about the same time that your mustache is growing in, hairs usually being to grow on the upper part of your cheeks and just below the center of your lower lip. Your sideburns may also grow at this time.

As you continue to mature, your facial hair will get thicker and darker in color. Your beard and mustache may be the same color as the hair on your head, or they may be a different color. You may find that by age eighteen, your beard and mustache are as full and thick as they're ever going to be. However, many men don't develop their full facial hair until ten years after they have completed puberty and reached their full adult height. Many a man finds that he can grow a thick beard or a bushy mustache and sideburns at age thirty, even though he hardly had any facial hair when he was in his teens or early twenties.

Shaving

Some grown men shave off their facial hair every day or even twice a day (if they have thick, fast-growing hair). Others will let their mustaches, sideburns, and/or beards grow and only trim them every once in a while to keep them neat. Still others just let their facial hair grow and only rarely, if ever, shave or trim it. It is a personal thing, a matter of individual taste.

Many of the men we talked to shaved when their facial hair first started to grow, even if later in life they decided not to shave. One mustached man said:

> I don't shave it now. When I was a teenager I did, though —because it was just these few scrawny hairs. It looked

pretty pathetic; kind of scraggly. It didn't look like a real mustache.

Phil, age 30

Another man said:

I don't shave anymore, just too lazy to shave every day. When I got that first peach fuzz, I shaved every day, religiously. It was kind of a macho thing. Also, I don't know if it's true or not, but I heard the more you shave, the faster your mustache and beard would grow in.

Ted, age 36

(By the way, Ted is probably right. Shaved hairs tend to grow back darker and thicker.)

A lot of the boys we talked to felt excited about shaving and looked upon shaving as a sign of growing up. Many boys wished they had as much facial hair as some of their friends had. One man told a funny story about this:

I ran around with my cousin, Albert, and his gang, who were all in their mid-twenties. I was, say, nineteen. Albert had a car, a Model-T, which was something—having a car that is—in those days. So it was really exciting for me to run around with these older guys. I wanted to look as old as them, so I'd get my mother's eyebrow pencil and color my mustache in, you know, to make me look more mature.

So we go to a dance, and afterward I'm smooching with this gal in the back seat of Albert's car, and my mustache smears off all over her face. Jeez, talk about embarrassing. I thought I'd never live it down!

Charlie, age 67

Getting their first razor was also a big event for some boys. Some bought these razors themselves; others got theirs as gifts. Some used their dad's razor at first:

When I first started shaving, I didn't say anything to anyone. I didn't want to buy one [a razor] and just leave it there in the bathroom 'cause I knew my family would just tease me to death about it. I really didn't have that much to shave. So I just used my dad's razor.

My sisters were starting to shave their legs, and they were using dad's razor, too. He'd get hopping mad 'cause he'd go to shave his face and the blade would be dull and nicked 'cause my sisters and I used it all the time. He'd cut his face all up and then he'd start hollerin', "Who's been using my razor?" My sisters and I would say, "Not me, not me!" Finally he went out and bought us all razors and told us, "You kids use my razor again and I'll kill you."

Sam, age 35

If you do start to shave, make sure that the blades of your razor are smooth and free of nicks, or you're apt to cut yourself. A dull blade can pull at your skin and irritate it, so make sure you've got a sharp one. But go easy—you can cut yourself with a sharp blade. Using soap or shaving cream will ease the pull or drag of the razor on your skin. There are also electric razors. You're a lot less likely to cut yourself with an electric razor, but some men don't like them. You might talk to your dad or another adult male to find out what he recommends for shaving.

UNDERARM HAIR AND PERSPIRATION

At about the same time that you start growing facial hair, you'll probably notice hair growing under your armpits. Occasionally, there's a boy who develops underarm hair before he begins to grow a mustache or even before he develops pubic hair. But for most boys, facial hair and underarm hair appear at about the same time.

Once you begin to grow underarm hair, or even before, you may notice that your underarms perspire (sweat) more, and that your perspiration has a different odor from when you were younger. You may also notice that other areas of your body, such as your genitals and your feet, have a different odor. Or you may notice that your hands tend to perspire and get rather clammy from time to time.

These changes happen because the testosterone from your testicles affects the sweat glands located in these areas of your body. It is all a natural, healthy part of growing up, but some teenagers worry about the smells and the increase in perspiration. Actually, it's not too surprising that some teenagers are concerned. Advertising agencies spend millions of dollars each year on TV commercials designed to make us worry about our body odors and whether or not we're "dry" enough. But if you're eating properly and are healthy, your body odor probably isn't offensive. Bathing or showering regularly and wearing freshly laundered clothes should keep you smelling clean and fresh. If you perspire quite a bit and this bothers you, you may find that wearing 100 percent cotton undershirts and shorts will help. Cotton is more absorbent than synthetic (man-made) materials. Wearing outer shirts and pants made of cotton or wool or other natural fibers may also help.

We all tend to perspire more when we're nervous. During puberty, this tendency may be even more noticeable. Lots of teenagers get clammy hands or break out in a sweat when they get uptight. This is perfectly normal and usually lessens after you reach your twenties. If you have this problem, it helps to remember that it is normal. Sometimes just admitting to yourself, "Yup, I'm feeling really nervous (or embarrassed or uptight) right now," will help you relax and perspire less.

Deodorants and Antiperspirants

If you are bothered by the odor or amount of your perspiration, you may want to use a deodorant and/or an antiperspirant. There are a number of these products on the market. They come in aerosol cans, non-aerosol sprays, sticks, creams, roll-ons—you name it. Some are "unscented," and some have a scent added to cover up the smell of the product. Some are advertised as being "a man's deodorant," but there generally isn't much difference between a so-called man's deodorant and a woman's deodorant.

Deodorants are aimed at covering up your body odor with the supposedly more pleasant odor of the deodorant. Antiperspirants also have a substance to dry up perspiration. The most effective antiperspirants have a substance called aluminum chlorohydrate. Some people think that the aluminum can soak through your skin and get into your bloodstream, and that this may be harmful. Other people disagree. You'll have to decide for yourself whether you want to use this kind of product.

Whatever you decide, be sure to read the label. Some products work best when you use them at bedtime rather than first thing in the morning. You may find that it is better not to put the deodorant or antiperspirant on just after you jump out of a hot shower. If you perspire after the shower, the deodorant/antiperspirant may just wash away. It might be better to let your body cool down a bit first.

With the way we've been going on about deodorants and perspiration here, you may be thinking, "Oh, wow, I'd better run right out and get some." Please remember, though, that body smells are natural and normal, and unless your odor or the amount of perspiration bothers you, it's not really necessary to use anything.

SKIN CHANGES

At the same time that your sweat glands are becoming more active, your body's oil glands are also working harder. As we explained in Chapter 2, more oil will be produced by the glands in your genital area, and this may make the skin of your penis and scrotum feel somewhat moist. The oil glands in your scalp may also start producing more. You may find that your hair gets more oily or greasy and that you have to shampoo it more often.

Pimples, Acne, and Other Skin Disturbances

The oil glands in your skin are also affected by the hormones your body starts making during puberty. Your skin becomes more oily, and for many boys and girls, this leads to skin problems like pimples. Some boys and girls have only mild problems with their skin; others have more severe problems; still others don't have problems at all. But eight out of every ten teenagers have at least mild skin problems, and boys seem to be even more susceptible than girls.

Pimples and other skin disturbances happen because the hormones, such as testosterone, that your body begins making during puberty cause your oil glands to make excess amounts of a substance called *sebum*. You have oil glands all over your skin. They are especially numerous on your face, neck, shoulders, upper chest, and back. Illustration 15 shows an oil gland. Sebum is made in the lower part of the gland and travels through the duct to the *pore*, the opening on the surface of your skin.

sebum (SEE-bum)

If you're producing a great deal of sebum, the pore may become clogged, and a blackhead may form. A lot of people think that blackheads are little particles of dirt trapped in the pores. This isn't true. Blackheads are black not from dirt but because the sebum and other substances produced by the glands sometimes turn black when they come in contact with the oxygen in the air.

Some boys and girls get whiteheads, which are also the result of sebum. The sebum gets trapped just below the surface of the skin and forms the small, raised whitish bumps we call whiteheads.

If blackheads are not removed, the sebum may continue to fill the duct. This may cause pressure, irritation, and inflammation. Germs can get in the duct and cause an infection. Whiteheads can also become inflamed and infected. Pimples—red bumps that may be filled with whitish pus and that many teenagers call "zits"—may develop. If you have a serious case of infected pimples, you may have a problem called *acne*. Acne can be very

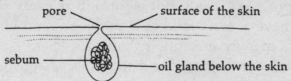

We have tiny oil glands just below the surface of our skin. These oil glands produce an oily substance called sebum.

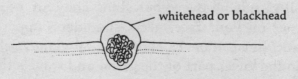

During puberty, our oil glands begin producing more sebum. If the pore, or opening, to the gland becomes blocked, a pimple may form.

Illustration 15. Oil gland

troublesome and may cause pitting or scarring of the skin.

Pimples and acne are often more of a problem for those who naturally tend to have more oily skin. The oiliness of your skin type, plus the increased oil you produce during puberty, combine to make you a candidate for these kinds of skin problems. If you have oily skin and acne during your teen years, you may find yourself wishing you had drier, less acne-prone skin. But when you're older, you may be glad to have oily skin, because this type of skin doesn't wrinkle as easily as dry skin does.

Acne also tends to "run in families," so if your parents or older brothers and sisters had acne, you may be more likely to develop it. Many doctors believe that eating certain foods—chocolate, salty foods like nuts and chips, and greasy foods—make a person more susceptible to acne. However, some doctors disagree. In one study, the amount of chocolate eaten didn't seem to have anything to do with acne. Still, if you find that certain foods give you pimples, it's best to avoid those foods.

Stress may also be a factor in acne. A lot of teens find that they "break out"—that is, get a lot of pimples —just before an important event—a dance, a big date, a game—that they're particularly nervous or excited about.

Although sunlight may have a beneficial effect on acne and help to "dry out" your skin, it may also aggravate the problem. If you live in a hot dry climate like that found in California, the sunshine may be helpful. However, hot humid (moist) climates, such as those of Hawaii or Florida, may make your acne even worse.

acne (AK-nee)

Some teens sit under a sunlamp to help dry out their acne and/or to get a tan. This isn't always a good idea. For one thing, sitting under a sunlamp can cause a severe sunburn, even if you only sit there for a minute more than the recommended time. While you're under the lamp, it may not seem like much is happening, so it's tempting to stay longer. All too often, this results in red, sunburned skin the next day. If you use a sunlamp, _follow the instructions carefully_. Another problem with sunlamps, or for that matter, with prolonged sunbathing, is that it can cause your skin to age before its time. People who have spent a lot of time in the sun or under sunlamps may be wrinkly and look like they're fifty or sixty by the time they're thirty. Overexposure to sunlight also increases your chances of getting skin cancer later in life. So be sure to go easy on the sun and tanning treatments.

Acne is most common between the ages of fourteen and seventeen, although it also happens to older and younger boys and girls. In boys, it tends to be worse during Stages 3 and 4 of genital development.

Some teens are troubled by acne for only a year or two. Then their oil glands adjust themselves to the hormones, their skin becomes less oily, and their acne and pimples clear up. Others have these problems throughout their teenage years. For a few boys and girls, acne continues to be a problem even after their teens.

The kids in my class generally want to know if there is anything they can do to prevent pimples or to cure acne. I explain that although there aren't any foolproof ways to prevent pimples, or any 100 percent effective cures for acne, there are some things that help many teens. Frequent shampoos will keep greasy, oily hair from adding to the oil on your skin. Washing the especially oily areas—your face, neck, shoulders, back, and upper chest—at least once a day may also help prevent pimples. Washing removes the oil from the surface of the skin and helps keep your pores open. Wash with hot water, which helps open your pores, and rinse with cold water to close the pores up again. Wiping with a pad soaked in isopropyl alcohol after you wash will remove any leftover oil and dirt. You can buy isopropyl alcohol for under fifty cents a bottle in a drugstore, and use cotton balls or pads. You can also buy special presoaked pads, but they're usually rather expensive. Go easy with the alcohol, though. It can remove too much oil and leave your skin too dry.

If you have especially oily skin, you may want to wash two or three times a day with ordinary soap. If you tend to get pimples, one of the antibacterial soaps sold in drugstores and pharmacies may help. (Ask the druggist to recommend one.) If you have pimples on your back, shower once or twice a day using an anti-bacterial soap and a back brush to scrub.

If you have blackheads, an abrasive soap or cleanser may help. (Again, ask your druggist to recommend one.) The abrasive in the soap often removes the blackheads and opens your pores. Be careful, though, because these soaps can irritate your skin. Don't use them more often than the instructions recommend. Also, black teens should *avoid* abrasives because their skin has a tendency to develop lighter or darker patches in the areas where they've used the abrasives.

Washing, even with antibacterial soaps or abrasives, isn't always enough to prevent pimples and doesn't do much to help acne. Occasionally, mild cases of acne can be cleared up by using medicated acne lotions and creams that are sold without prescription. If these medications and the washing routines we've described don't take care of your problem and you're really bothered by acne, you should see a dermatologist, a doctor who specializes in skin problems.

A lot of times, parents say, "Oh, it's not that bad," or "Leave it alone, you'll outgrow it." But if you take the time to explain to your parents how much your skin problems bother you, they'll probably listen. If your family doesn't have medical insurance or coverage that will pay for the dermatologist, you may find that your parents are concerned about the cost. Many families don't have money to spend on doctor's visits unless you're actually sick. If money is a problem, perhaps you can find some odd jobs to earn enough to pay for the dermatologist yourself. You might call some dermatologists; your family doctor or local medical association, which is listed in the yellow pages under "Physicians," can give you names of dermatologists in your area. Ask how much the doctor charges. Some doctors will let you work out a payment plan by which you give a little money each week until your bill is paid up.

What can a dermatologist do for you? Well, that depends. If blackheads are a problem, the doctor can use a device called a comedo extractor to remove the blackheads. The comedo extractor (*comedo* is the scientific term for blackhead) exerts pressure on the skin and causes the blackhead to pop out of the pore, thus unclogging the duct. The area around the blackhead may be a little red for a while, but unlike squeezing or "popping" your blackheads with your fingers, the comedo extractor won't cause scars. You should never pop your blackheads or pimples because you might wind up with permanent scars or pits. The extractor is used only on blackheads. Once you've got an actual pimple, using the extractor may cause more harm than good.

comedo (KOM-i-DOUGH)

The dermatologist can also prescribe drugs that are more effective than the medications you can buy without a doctor's prescription. For example, in certain cases, the dermatologist may prescribe a drug called tetracycline. Tetracycline kills germs and can fight the infections that often start in clogged pores and lead to acne. This drug also cuts down on the amount of sebum your oil glands produce. For some teens, tetracycline works miracles and completely cures their acne. However, you should only use it according to your doctor's orders because in some people it can cause problems, such as upset stomach and increased sensitivity to sunlight (sunburns). These and other side effects are usually pretty mild but you must follow your doctor's orders carefully.

If tetracycline doesn't work for you (and it *doesn't* work for everyone), your doctor may prescribe other treatments. He or she might, for instance, prescribe a gel or cream containing retinoic acid. This medication is effective when applied on the face, but it doesn't work on other areas, like your shoulders or back. For the first week or so, your face may look even worse, but then your skin will usually peel and look better. There are also other treatments a dermatologist can prescribe, so if you're troubled by skin problems, it may be worth your while to see a dermatologist.

Stretch Marks
Some boys and girls develop stretch marks, purplish or white lines on their skin, during puberty. This is fairly rare, but it does occur. It happens because the skin is stretched too much during rapid growth, and it loses its

tetracycline (TET-reh-SIGH-clean)
retinoic (reh-tin-OH-ic)

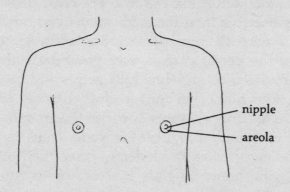

Illustration 16. The breast. In the center of each breast is a small raised part called the "nipple," which is surrounded by a ring of skin called the "areola."

elasticity, or stretchiness. (Other things, such as taking certain medications, being pregnant, or gaining a lot of weight can also cause stretch marks.) Many times these marks will fade or get less noticeable as a person gets older, but they may never disappear completely.

BREAST CHANGES

We usually think of breast change as something that happens to girls, because during puberty their breasts begin to grow and develop (as we explain in Chapter 6). Although boys' breasts don't change as dramatically as girls' do, there are certain changes in your breasts that you may notice at this time in your life. For one thing, the *areola,* the ring of colored flesh around your nipple, may get wider and darker in color (see Illustration 16). The nipple may also get a bit larger.

areola (ah-ree-OH-la)

You may notice that your breasts feel tender or sore. Many boys notice a flat, buttonlike bump under one or both nipples. If this happens to you and you don't know that it's perfectly normal, it can be a bit scary. As one man told us:

I had these bumps under my nipples. I thought I had cancer or something.

Harold, age 34

Even though these lumps can be uncomfortable, or even downright painful, they aren't anything to worry about. It's just a reaction to the new hormones your body is making. Eventually, the lumps and soreness will go away. It's perfectly normal and not a sign that you have cancer or any other disease. (Men, by the way, only rarely get cancer of the breast, and young boys almost *never* do.)

Out of every 100 boys between 50 and 85 of them will experience some swelling of the breasts as they go through puberty. In some boys, this swelling is more noticeable than in others. The swelling may be accompanied by soreness. There may also be lumps, of the type described above, under one or both breasts. This swelling can last from one year to a year and a half.

Although this, too, is a normal and natural change— and even though it happens to more than half of the boys going through puberty—boys really worry about it. Over the years, I've gotten a lot of questions about this in the question box in my class. Boys worry because they think they're going to start to grow breasts and turn into girls or something. One man who had quite a bit of breast swelling during puberty told us how he felt:

It was like I was growing breasts, and mine were even bigger than some of the girls'! I got teased about it all the time. I was really afraid that I was turning into a girl, that someone had made this big mistake and I really *was* a girl. I thought my penis was maybe going to fall off or something and I'd grow breasts and have to wear a bra. I'd heard all sorts of wild stories about boys who turned out to be women and had breasts *and* penises. But I didn't know anyone I could ask about it.

By the time I was in high school, my chest looked normal. My breasts had gone away. I wish I'd known that it was going to be okay because I really worried about it for a while.

Tom, age 40

You may also notice that your breasts are swelling, and you may have the same kind of worries Tom had. Relax—we promise, you won't turn into a girl! Within about a year to a year and a half, the swelling will go away. If you've heard stories like the ones Tom mentioned you may have wondered if they're true. It is true that some people are born with both male and female sex organs. Such people are called *hermaphrodites*.

Hermaphrodites have both testicles and ovaries on the inside of their bodies. On the outside, a hermaphrodite might have a penis, a man's body build, and a beard, but breasts like a woman's. A hermaphrodite can also look like a woman, with a curvy body shape, breasts, and no beard, but have a penis instead of a vulva, or have the inner and outer lips of a vulva but a penis instead of a clitoris. There are any number of different ways that a hermaphrodite might look, and sometimes their genital organs don't quite look like those of either sex.

When I explain to the kids in my class about hermaphrodites, I usually see a few kids gulping and look-

hermaphrodites (her-MAF-row-dites)

ing very nervous or worried. Boys whose breasts have been swelling or who have been slow to develop start to worry, "Oh, no, maybe I'm a hermaphrodite!" Some of the girls who have been slow in developing look worried too.

I tell them not to worry. For one thing, hermaphroditism is *very*, *very* rare. Besides, if they were hermaphrodites they'd already know it. It is usually obvious right when a baby is born. (Nowadays doctors are able to do special plastic surgery operations on the sex organs on the outside of the body so the child will grow up looking like a normal male or female, depending on which sex is most appropriate in that particular child's case. So, today most hermaphrodites grow up looking quite normal, though their reproductive organs usually do not work right; they may have to take certain hormones and they usually aren't able to have children.)

VOICE CHANGES

Another change you may notice as you go through puberty is that your voice becomes lower and deeper. This happens because testosterone causes your *larynx*, or voice box (the part of your throat that contains your vocal cords), to grow larger. Your vocal cords get thicker and longer, and this changes the tone of your voice. Voice changes usually happen when a boy is about fourteen or fifteen, but they may happen earlier or later than this.

For some boys, this voice change happens without their really noticing it:

larynx (LARR-inks)

I didn't realize that my voice had changed, except that people stopped thinking I was my mom or my sister when I'd answer the phone.

Bill, age 19

For some boys, the change in their voices is more sudden and noticeable:

My throat was sore for about a month or so, kind of scratchy. I thought I just had some kind of sore throat. My voice was kind of froggy. I was always going ahem, ahem—you know, how you clear your throat. Afterward I noticed my voice was deeper than before.

Phil, age 17

Some boys experience what is called "cracking" of their voices as they're going through this voice change. They'll be talking in a normal voice and all of a sudden their voice will get very high and squeaky. A lot of boys found this cracking one of the most embarrassing things about going through puberty. As one man explained:

I'd finally get up my nerve to call a girl on the phone and ask her for a date. I'd say, "Hi, Susie," or whatever her name was, "this is John," and my voice would be just fine. I'd sound perfectly cool. Then I'd say, "Would you like to go to the movies?"—and right in the middle my voice would go all high and funny. It would sound like it was Minnie Mouse talking.

John, age 36

Another man said:

Really, it was the most embarrassing thing. It seemed like it happened about all the time. I'd try to control my voice and never get really excited or happy-sounding. Anytime I got nervous and excited, that's when it would happen. I tried not to get too emotional, but of course I did. I never really got control over it. Finally, after a year or maybe it was two years, it stopped happening.

Tyrone, age 28

Your voice may change suddenly and dramatically or it may happen without your really noticing it. Like John and Tyrone, your voice may crack and you may feel embarrassed about it, although there's no real reason to be embarrassed, because people know it's just a part of growing up. Eventually, though, your voice will "settle down" and you'll find yourself sounding more adult.

PUBERTY IS NOT A DISEASE!

It usually takes an entire class period for us to cover the changes we've been talking about in this chapter. The kids in my class are curious about these things, and they often have a lot of questions. Most of them agree that knowing about things like sore or swollen breasts, pimples, stretch marks, and cracking voices helps you to deal with them if they happen to you. Still, hearing about all of them at once can be a bit overwhelming. As one boy put it:

I'm not sure I'm exactly looking forward to all these things happening to me. Puberty is beginning to sound like some kind of disease!

Puberty definitely isn't a disease. The changes we've described in this chapter and in other parts of this book are natural and healthy. They're a normal part of growing up and becoming a man. Still, when we start focusing on things like perspiration, pimples, cracking voices, and so on, puberty can start to sound like just one hassle after another. By the end of the class in which we cover these things, I can see that some of the kids are starting to think that puberty sounds like more trouble than it's worth! So I tell them, "Hey, don't get discouraged!"

First of all, the problem things don't happen to everyone. Not everyone has pimples, a voice that cracks, or swollen, sore breasts. For most kids, the physical changes of puberty happen without any difficulties. And even for those who do have some problems, it's not such a big deal. So your voice cracks. Even if it's embarrassing, no one ever died of embarrassment.

Sometimes, spending a whole class period—or, in the case of this book, a whole chapter—on these problems can give you a distorted picture. It can make them loom larger or seem more important than they really are. So at the end of the class, I ask everyone to make a list of the five things they like best about going through puberty and growing up. Here are some of the things the boys in my classes have come up with.

more privileges	getting my braces off
getting to stay out later	getting a job
being more my own boss	dating
driving a car	getting into R-rated movies
new friends	having my body get stronger
new school	going to parties
more respect	having my own money
more allowance	joining the team in high school
making my own decisions (sometimes)	going to college
hanging out with the older guys	

Perhaps you'd like to take a few minutes to make a list of your own, to help yourself remember that puberty is a lot more than just pimples and perspiration!

CHAPTER 5

Ejaculation, Orgasms, Erections, Masturbation, and Wet Dreams

Way back in Chapter 1, we talked about ejaculation. We explained that when a man and a woman are having sexual intercourse, the man may ejaculate his sperm into the woman's vagina. When this happens, muscles in his genital area contract and sperm are pumped out of his testicles, through a hollow tube in the center of the penis, and out the opening in the center of the glans (the "tip" or "head") of his penis.

Men don't always ejaculate when they're having sex, but usually they do. A man or boy may ejaculate at other times too, even if he's not having sexual intercourse. In fact, boys usually have their first ejaculations around their fourteenth birthdays, long before most of them have started having sexual intercourse. In this

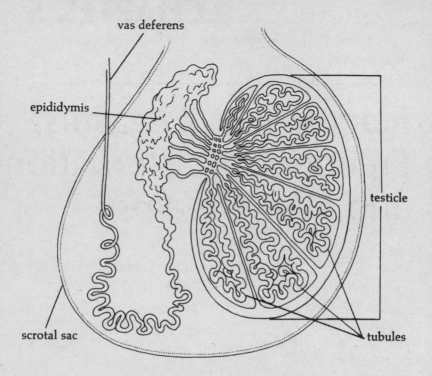

Illustration 17. Cross section of the scrotum. This drawing shows the inside of a scrotal sac. The sperm are made in the tubules, inside the testicle. Then they travel to the epididymis, where they ripen. From there, they move through the vas deferens, up into the main part of the body.

chapter, we'll talk about the things other than sexual intercourse that can cause you to ejaculate, and we'll also talk about your first ejaculation.

THE INSIDE STORY

In order to understand ejaculation, it helps to have some idea of how the sex organs on the inside of the body work. Illustration 17 shows a cross section of one of the scrotal sacs. (If this drawing looks a bit confusing to you or you've forgotten how cross-section drawings work, you might want to take another look at Illustration 5 on page 19.)

The Testicles

As you may recall, the testicles, or testes, rest inside the scrotum. Each testicle is made up of separate compartments. We couldn't draw small enough to get them all in this illustration, but there are about two hundred and fifty of these little compartments in each testicle. Inside each compartment are tiny, thread-like tubes called *tubules*, which are coiled up and packed tightly. If you unwound all the tubules in your testicles and stretched them out end to end, they'd stretch the length of several football fields.

During puberty, a boy begins to make sperm inside these tubules, and he continues to make fresh sperm every day for the rest of his life. Sperm production slows down a bit in old age, but until then, a male makes millions of sperm each day.

Sperm are alive. When they're fully mature, they look like tadpoles, with rounded bodies and tiny tails. Of course, real sperm are much smaller than the critter you

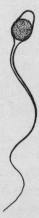

Illustration 18. A sperm

see in Illustration 18. In fact, it would take five hundred sperm, lined up end to end, to cover a distance of one inch. You can't even see a sperm unless you use a microscope.

The Epididymis

After the sperm are made, they travel from the tubules inside the testicle to the *epididymis*, a special compartment attached to the testicle. The epididymis is also composed of tiny tubes. It is here, inside these tubes, that the sperm ripen into mature sperm. It takes the sperm about four to six weeks to travel through the epididymis, during which time they complete their ripening.

The Vas Deferens

Once they're fully mature, the sperm are ready to travel out of the scrotal sac and up into the body, where they are stored until you ejaculate. To get from the scrotum to the main part of your body, the sperm travel through a tube called the *vas deferens* (also called the vas or sperm duct). You have two sperm ducts, one for each testicle. Each one is between fourteen and eighteen inches long. You can only see the bottom part of one vas in Illustration 17. But if you look at Illustration 19, you'll see that the rest of the vas runs up out of the scrotum and into the main part of your body.

Perhaps you've wondered why the testicles and scrotum hang down, outside and away from the main part of your body. As one boy in my class put it:

> Why do they dangle down there like that where they can get hit and knocked around? Why aren't they tucked up inside your body where they'd be safe?

epididymis (eh-pih-DIH-dih-miss)
vas (VAS) *deferens* (DEF-eh-renz)

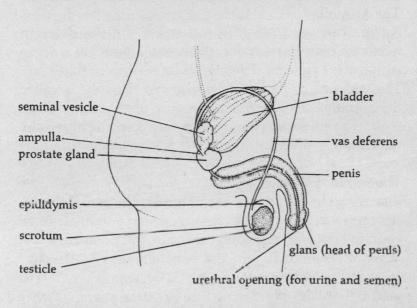

seminal vesicle

ampulla

prostate gland

epididymis

scrotum

testicle

bladder

vas deferens

penis

glans (head of penis)

urethral opening (for urine and semen)

Illustration 19. Cross section of the sex organs on the inside of the male body

It's a good question, and there's a good answer. In order for your testicles to make sperm, they have to be at exactly the right temperature. The right temperature is a little *lower* than the temperature of the rest of your body. If your testicles were up inside your body, they'd get too hot to make sperm. So, instead, they hang down in the scrotal sac, away from your body. This way air can circulate around them and keep them cool. In cold weather or when you jump into a cold pool, the scrotum tightens up, bringing your testicles closer to your body for extra warmth. In hot weather, after a hot bath, or when you have a fever, the scrotum relaxes and hangs lower so that your testicles are farther away from your body and can stay cool.

The Ampulla

As you can see from Illustration 19, the vas deferens winds up over the bladder, the hollow, pouchlike organ where urine collects. Then the tube widens or flares out. The widened or flared-out portion of the tube is called the *ampulla*. The ampulla is a sort of "sperm storage tank" or reservoir, where sperm are kept until they're ejaculated.

The Seminal Vesicles

Just at the lower part of the ampulla, the *seminal vesicles* connect up to the vas. You have two seminal vesicles, but you can only see one in Illustration 19. *Seminal* refers to sperm, and *vesicle* means "little sac," so together the words mean "little sperm sac." The seminal vesicles got their name because scientists once thought that sperm were stored there until they were ejaculated. We now know that sperm are stored in the ampulla, but the name still sticks.

Even though they don't store sperm, the seminal vesicles have an important job. They make the white sticky fluid called *semen*, or seminal fluid, that spurts out of your penis when you ejaculate. Mixed in with this fluid are millions of sperm from your ampulla. But sperm are so tiny that they account for only about one-tenth of the teaspoon of milky fluid that comes out when you ejaculate. The other nine-tenths of your ejaculate is composed mostly of fluid from the seminal vesicles.

Semen

Semen is very powerful stuff. You know how during a game football players drink Gatorade, which is packed

ampulla (am-PUL-ah or am-POOL-ah)
seminal (SEM-eh-nul) *vesicles* (VES-eh-kuls)
semen (SEA-men)

full of sugar and vitamins, to give them an instant energy boost? Well, semen is like Gatorade for sperm. Just before ejaculation, the seminal vesicles release semen into the ampulla. The sperm are zapped by a shot of the sugar-rich semen, which gives them a big energy boost.

Until the seminal fluid mixes with the sperm, the sperm are sort of sluggish and slow-moving. They hardly move their tails. They don't even have enough energy to get around by themselves.

Luckily, the walls of the vas deferens have muscles that work something like the muscles in your throat. These muscles contract, and, with the help of tiny little hairs, they sweep the sperm up the tube of the vas deferens into the ampulla. Otherwise, the sluggish sperm would never get themselves out of the scrotum.

Once the sperm get a shot of semen, they start whipping their tails around like wild and moving all over the place. Sperm really need this energy boost. They have quite a long journey to make in order to get to the ovum and fertilize it. After the sperm and semen are ejaculated from the man's penis into the woman's vagina, the sperm have to travel to the top of the woman's vagina and through the narrow opening there that leads to her uterus. Then they have to travel the whole length of the woman's uterus and halfway up her fallopian tube in order to meet up with and fertilize the ovum. (Look back at Illustration 6, page 20, if you don't remember what these body parts look like.) And the sperm have to move quickly in order to get to the ovum while it's still nice and fresh. So the sperm are "running" the whole way.

Altogether it's only a distance of about six inches that the sperm have to travel, which doesn't sound like much. Remember, though, sperm are less than one five-hundredth of an inch long. Six inches to a sperm would be like four miles to a man. You'd certainly need an energy boost if you were going to run four miles at top speed!

The Prostate Gland

The prostate gland, which lies below the ampulla and seminal vesicles, is ring-shaped. A number of tubes, including the vas deferens, run through the center of this ring. The prostate gland also adds some fluid to the semen. When a man ejaculates, the prostate contracts and tightens up, squeezing on the vas. This helps push the sperm and the other seminal fluids (that is, the semen) into the tube in the center of the penis that is called the *urethra*.

The Urethra

The urethra is yet another tube. (Seems like you're just full of tubes, doesn't it?) As you can see from looking at Illustration 19, the urethra is in the center of the penis. It is cushioned by the soft, spongy tissue on the inside of the penis. The sperm and seminal fluid travel through the urethra and spurt out the opening in the center of the glans, or head, of the penis during ejaculation. Urine from the bladder also travels along the urethra when you urinate (pee). The tube from the bladder and the vas deferens both connect up with the urethra.

When I tell the kids in my class that urine and sperm both use the urethra to get out of the body, someone usually blurts out, "Oh, gross!" Even if no one says anything, I can see from their wrinkled-up noses and the looks on their faces that many kids think this sounds pretty disgusting.

prostate (PROS-tate)
urethra (you-REE-thra)

But, really, there's nothing gross or disgusting about it. Urine is just another liquid, and unless you have an infection, it doesn't have any disease-causing germs in it. Semen is perfectly clean too. Besides, sperm and urine can't travel through the urethra tube at the same time. When you're about to ejaculate, there's a valve at the bottom of the bladder that closes off so that urine can't get into the urethra when sperm is about to travel through there. Also, just before you ejaculate, two small glands in the area release a little bit of liquid into the urethra to flush it out and neutralize any acidy urine that might still be in there. (Sperm are sensitive to acids, so it's necessary to neutralize any acid in the urethra before the sperm travels through it.)

Even though I try to explain all this really carefully, I almost always get a question about it in the Everything You Ever Wanted to Know question box at the end of the class. Usually, the question has something to do with whether or not a man can urinate and ejaculate at the same time. Or, as one kid wrote, "Can a man piss inside a woman's vagina?"

I must admit, when I first got this question, I didn't quite understand it. I thought the kid who wrote it must have been putting me on. (Some kids in my classes do try to put me on, especially at the beginning of the year. They'll put questions in the box that have lots of so-called dirty words or are really gross, hoping to embarrass me when I read them out loud. But they soon give up on this because, as you may have guessed, I don't get embarrassed very easily, at least not by dirty words or questions about sex.)

At any rate, I finally figured out what the kid who wrote the question was getting at. He or she was wondering if a man could by accident urinate (piss) instead of ejaculate during sexual intercourse. Actually, when you think of how all those tubes are connected up, it's a pretty logical question. But the answer is no. When a male is about to ejaculate, the valve I mentioned earlier closes up. It seals off the bladder, and urine can't come through the urethra during ejaculation.

EJACULATION AND ORGASM

When a male ejaculates, the muscles around the prostate gland, as well as the muscles in the penis and surrounding area, contract. These muscle contractions, or spasms, force most of the sperm out of the ampulla. The sperm and semen mix together and are pushed into the urethra. They're propelled along the urethra and come spurting out the opening in the glans, or tip, of the penis. The semen usually comes out in three or four spurts. In all, about a teaspoon or so of white, creamy, milky semen comes out of the penis during ejaculation.

The feeling that you get when all these muscles are contracting and semen is spurting out of your penis is called *orgasm*. It is possible to ejaculate without having an orgasm, but most of the time a male does have one when he ejaculates. Slang terms for having an orgasm include "coming," "climaxing," and "getting off."

It's a bit difficult to describe exactly what an orgasm feels like. For one thing, it feels different to different people. Also, the feeling of an orgasm may differ from one time to the next. Sometimes the orgasm may be really strong and involve not just the penis and other sex organs but the whole body. At other times, the orgasm may be less intense, and the feeling seems to center around the penis and the genital area.

orgasm (OR-gaz-um)

When a male is about to have an orgasm, his penis is stiff and erect. The skin on his scrotum gets tighter and thicker as the scrotum draws up close to his body. His heart starts beating harder and his breathing gets deeper and heavier. The skin on his face or chest or other parts of his body may get flushed and reddish in color. This is called the "sex flush." His nipples may become deeper in color and stiffer and may stand out more. The muscles around his anus may tighten up. A drop or two of clear or milky white fluid may appear at the tip of the penis. The opening in the head, or glans, of the penis may become more slit-like, and the glans may become a deeper, more purplish or red color.

As the orgasm is about to begin, the man may be aware of all these changes (the increase in heartbeat, the heavier breathing, the changes in the glans), but often the feeling is so intense that he is totally involved only in the feeling. The changes may happen without his being consciously aware of them.

During the actual orgasm, the muscles contract and the semen comes out in three or four spurts that usually happen within less than a second of one another. These spurts may be followed by a series of six to fifteen other muscle spasms. The whole orgasm normally lasts about ten seconds. The feeling is so intense, though, that it often seems longer.

After the orgasm, the heartbeat and breathing gradually return to normal. The testicles and scrotum loosen up. The penis gets soft again. All of this may take just a few seconds, or it may take a half hour or so. Afterward, men often feel really relaxed, and they may be sleepy. Other men are ready to have another orgasm right away. Usually, though, there's a period of time that must pass—anywhere from a few minutes to a half hour, several hours, or a day or so—before a man is ready to have another orgasm. Generally, the older a man gets, the more time it takes before he's ready to have another orgasm.

As we say, it's a little difficult to explain how an orgasm feels, but most people agree that it's a super good feeling. We asked the men we interviewed to describe it, and many said things like "great," "terrific," "beautiful," or other simple, one-word answers. Most had trouble putting it into words, saying things like, "There's just no words to describe it," or "It's not something you can explain." Some men, however, were able to give a description. One man gave a description that other men seemed to think was pretty good. Here's what he said:

> Well, it feels like there's a sort of neat sensation in my genitals and body that builds up and then goes off, a sort of wave of good sensual feeling throughout the whole body. The spurting part, when the semen is actually coming out, is a jerky kind of thing. It's not really all that great a feeling, but the waves of the sensual feeling are timed with pulses of the spurt, which does feel great. Afterward, I feel tingling and then relaxed all over.
>
> Will, age 46

ERECTIONS

Before a male has an ejaculation or an orgasm, his penis gets stiff and hard, or at least semi-hard (halfway, or a little bit, hard). As you may recall from Chapter 1, this is called having an erection, or, in slang terms, a "boner" or a "hard-on." (You don't have an ejaculation every time you have an erection, however, just sometimes.)

During an erection, the blood passageways in the spongy tissue on the inside of the penis fill with blood.

This causes the penis to get stiff and hard and stand out from the body. Of course, there's always *some* blood inside your penis, just as there's always some blood in every part of your body. Our hearts are continually pumping blood throughout our bodies, and this flow of blood helps keep each part of us healthy and strong. But when the penis is erect there's more blood than usual in it. The muscles at the base of the penis tighten up and close off the passageways that normally allow blood to flow out of the penis, trapping the blood and causing the penis to swell and become larger and harder.

An erection can happen very quickly. In just a few seconds, the penis may go from being completely soft and floppy to being quite hard. Or an erection may happen more slowly and gradually. Sometimes the penis gets *really* hard and stiff. At other times, the penis may get only semi-hard.

When the penis gets erect, it also gets longer and wider. It may get darker in color. The scrotum and testicles may pull up tighter and closer to the body. The blood vessels (blood passageways) on the surface of the penis may bulge out, and the skin covering the blood vessels may turn bluish or darker in color.

Some penises are quite straight when they are erect, but many are slightly curved or bent. Sometimes the erect penis stands out at a right angle from the body, but usually it points upward. It may even stick practically straight up (see Illustration 20).

Erections happen for all sorts of reasons. Stroking or touching the penis or the scrotum often causes an erection. The friction of your pants rubbing against your penis can cause one. Sometimes the penis becomes erect even though it has not been touched or rubbed. At times, a male may have an erection when he needs to urinate, or he may wake up in the morning with an erection.

Thinking "sexy" thoughts—that is, thinking about having sex, about being sexual, about your sex organs, or just about sex in general—may cause an erection. But sometimes males have erections even though they are not thinking about sex at all. Getting nervous or excited about something can cause an erection. Warm, nice feelings can cause one. In fact, erections sometimes happen when you are not thinking about anything in particular.

Males have erections, from time to time, throughout their whole lives. Even tiny babies have erections. Many boys find that once they start puberty, they have erections more frequently than they did before. They often have what we call "spontaneous erections." Spontaneous erections happen spontaneously—that is, "all by themselves"—even though the penis has not been stroked or touched. They can happen anywhere, at any

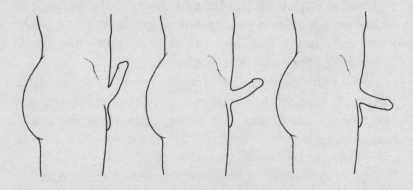

Illustration 20. Erections. The erect penis may stick out at various angles or may stand practically straight up.

spontaneous (spon-TAY-knee-us)

time. As we said, they may happen when you are thinking about sex or girls, when you get excited or nervous, or even when you are not feeling any particular way or thinking about anything in particular.

Not all boys notice that they start to have more erections than ever before as they are going through puberty. But many boys do. It is normal if you do and normal if you don't.

Boys who do have erections more frequently during puberty may have them quite often or only once in a while. The boys and men we interviewed for this book were very different in this way. Some rarely, if ever, had spontaneous erections. Others had them once a month; others once or twice a week. Still others had erections ten or twelve times a day.

The boys and men we talked to were often embarrassed when they had spontaneous erections. One boy in my class told a story that went something like this:

I was on the beach wearing my BVs [a bikini kind of bathing suit made out of thin, nylon material], and I saw this really curvy girl lying on her towel. My penis got hard and I had to run into the ocean so no one would see.

Another said:

Yeah, I get erections sometimes when I'm out running. That's how come I always wear a pair of gym shorts over my sweat pants. You get a hard-on and it sticks out like a tent pole in those baggy sweats.

One man remembered how it was for him:

It would happen any old time. I'd be at school, standing in the hall or something, and bingo, I'd have a hard-on. I'd shuffle my school books around and try and hold them in front of me so no one could see. It was really embarrassing.

Joe, age 32

Many told stories about getting erections when they had to get up in front of the class:

> I had to give a speech one time in public-speaking class. I had this really funny speech, and I'm standing there doing it and I get this big hard-on. I didn't know if everyone was laughing at my speech or at my hard-on.
>
> Tyrone, age 28

If you start to notice that you're having more erections as you're going through puberty, it helps to know that it's perfectly normal, that other boys are experiencing the same thing, and that your erections probably aren't as noticeable to other people as they are to you.

ONCE YOU HAVE AN ERECTION

Once you have an erection, one of two things will happen. First of all, the erection may go away all by itself. It may take a few seconds, a few minutes, or even a half hour or so before your penis is completely soft again. But after a while the muscles at the base of your penis will relax, allowing the extra blood that was trapped in the penis to flow back out so that the penis becomes soft and floppy again.

The second thing that can happen is that you will ejaculate and/or have an orgasm, after which the muscles at the base of the penis will relax and the penis will become soft again. As we explained, one thing that can cause a male to have an orgasm and to ejaculate is sexual intercourse. During sexual intercourse, the man puts his erect (or at least semi-erect) penis into the woman's vagina. As you may recall from Chapter 1, the vagina is a hollow organ. Normally, the vagina is like a collapsed balloon with no air in it; but it is very expandable, so the penis can fit right in there (see Illustration 21). The vagina fits snugly and tightly around

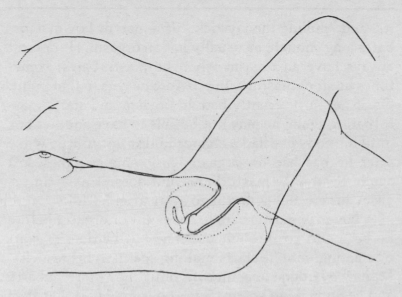

Illustration 21. Penis in vagina

the penis. During intercourse, a man moves his penis around in the vagina, which stimulates the nerves in the penis. When the penis is sufficiently stimulated, the man usually ejaculates. It's possible to ejaculate without having an orgasm. It's also possible to have an orgasm without ejaculating. But usually when a man is having sexual intercourse, he both ejaculates *and* has an orgasm. Soon afterward, his penis becomes soft again.

MASTURBATION

Another thing that can cause a male to ejaculate and/or have an orgasm is masturbation. *Masturbation* means "deliberate touching or stroking of the sex organs." Slang terms for masturbating include "jacking off," "playing with yourself," "beating your meat," "doing

masturbation (mass-tur-BAY-shun)

it," and "pulling the joystick." If a man or boy masturbates long enough, he usually has an orgasm. He doesn't always have an orgasm when he masturbates; sometimes he stops masturbating before he gets to that point. Or, if he's just recently had an orgasm and starts masturbating again, he may not be able to have another one until his body has had a chance to rest up. A little while after he has had an orgasm, his penis becomes soft again. Even if he masturbates and doesn't have an orgasm, his erection will still go away after a while.

A boy may masturbate to the point of orgasm before he begins to go through puberty, but he doesn't start ejaculating until he starts making sperm in his testicles. Many boys don't masturbate until they start puberty and begin making sperm. Such boys may find that they have their first orgasm at the same time that they have their first ejaculation.

The first ejaculation usually happens around the age of thirteen or fourteen. But some boys ejaculate before this, and others don't have ejaculations until they're fifteen and older. For some boys, the first ejaculation happens as a result of masturbating. For others, the first ejaculation happens in their sleep. This is called having a wet dream. We'll explain more about wet dreams later in this chapter, but for now we want to talk more about masturbation. Kids usually have lots of questions about masturbation, and here are answers to some of those questions.

Do most boys masturbate?
Yes, most boys (and men, too) masturbate. Not all do, though. It's normal if you do and normal if you don't.

Some men start to masturbate when they're kids and continue throughout their lives. Some start during

masturbates (MASS-tur-baits)

puberty. Some don't start until they're older. And there are some who never masturbate.

People sometimes think that the only men who masturbate are those who haven't started having sexual intercourse yet. They get the idea that once you start having sex, you stop masturbating. Not true. Many married men and also unmarried men, even if they're having sexual intercourse regularly, still masturbate.

Do girls masturbate?
Yes, girls and women also masturbate. Women don't, of course, ejaculate sperm like men do, but their genitals may feel very wet when they masturbate. This is because glands in the vulva and vagina give off fluids when a female becomes sexually aroused. Some women's glands produce a sudden gush of this fluid just as they're having an orgasm, but this is not an ejaculation of the type men have.

According to studies done by sex researchers, boys are more likely to masturbate than girls. But many of these studies were done ten or twenty years ago. Today, it's considered more acceptable for girls to know about and talk about their bodies, so many experts feel that nowadays the number of girls who masturbate may be much higher.

How often do boys masturbate?
This depends on the boy. Some masturbate several times a day; some once or twice a day; some once or twice a week. Some boys masturbate more often or less often than this, and some never masturbate.

Is masturbation bad for you?
No, masturbation is not in any way harmful. Back in your grandmother and grandfather's day, people

thought that all sorts of horrible things would happen if you masturbated. Masturbation was supposed to cause warts on your nose, hair to grow on the palms of your hands, pale skin, pimples, wet and clammy hands, blindness, softening of the brain, idiocy, and insanity (to mention just a few problems). Nowadays we know that none of these things is true. (If they were, there would be an awful lot of blind, insane idiots around.)

Even though people no longer believe these old stories, the idea that masturbation might be harmful or just not good for you still lingers on. Some people think that masturbating too much will cause you to "run out of" or "use up" all your sperm. But, as you know from reading this book, your body is constantly making millions of new sperm each day. There's just no way you could run out. Other people think that masturbating too much will somehow hurt your penis or sex organs. Again, this isn't true. If you masturbate and ejaculate a whole lot, your penis might get sore from all the rubbing, but other than this soreness, masturbating cannot hurt your body. In fact, it's just not possible for you to masturbate and ejaculate too much. Your body sets its own limits. If a boy is masturbating a great deal, after a while his penis just won't get erect anymore. He'll have to rest for a while before he can get an erection again.

Is it all right to imagine things when you masturbate?
Many people like to imagine things that make them feel more excited as they are masturbating. Imagining or pretending that something is happening is called daydreaming or fantasizing. We daydream and fantasize about all sorts of things. We might, for instance, daydream about being a major league football player or a rock star. When our daydreams are about sexual things, we call them sexual fantasies. Almost everyone has sex-

ual fantasies. We may have them while we're masturbating and at other times too. Sexual fantasies can be a rich and varied way of experimenting with your sexual self. Sometimes, the things we fantasize about are things we might actually like to do someday; other times we fantasize about things that we'd feel embarrassed or even bad about if we actually did them.

Some people worry that there might be something weird about their sexual fantasies. If you've ever been concerned about this, you can relax. Human beings (both males *and* females) have sexual fantasies about all sorts of things. If you think you're the only one who's ever had a particular fantasy—you're wrong. We guarantee that there are plenty of other people who've had almost the exact same fantasy.

Can masturbation affect your athletic performance?
In general, masturbating won't affect your athletic ability. Some athletic coaches think that it's a good idea for boys to masturbate before a big game. Masturbating is a way of relieving tension and is very relaxing. But there are some coaches who think that athletes perform better when they're somewhat tense and not completely relaxed, so they tell their teams to lay off masturbating or having sexual intercourse for a few days before a big game. If you're an athlete, you'll have to decide for yourself what works best for you.

Will masturbating a lot when you're young affect your sex life when you're older?
Some people think that if you masturbate a whole lot when you're young, you'll learn to like it so much that you won't enjoy sexual intercourse as much when you're older. This isn't true. In fact, most experts agree that masturbating is a way of rehearsing for your adult

sex life. By masturbating, you learn how your own body responds and what gives you the most pleasure. When you do begin to have sex, you are knowledgeable about what you like, about what "turns you on." If you know this about yourself, it's that much easier to tell your sex partner what you like and/or don't like and how your partner can help increase your sexual pleasure.

It is true that many men find that they have more physically intense orgasms from masturbation than from intercourse. (This doesn't necessarily mean that they *like* masturbation more than intercourse, because intercourse involves touching, holding, and being intimate with another person. That makes it a very different kind of experience than masturbating.) However, other men find that the orgasms they experience during intercourse are more intense than those they have during masturbation. Still others don't find any difference in intensity.

As you grow older, you may find that masturbating provides the most intense orgasms, that sexual intercourse does, or that both things provide equally intense orgasms. Regardless, how much or how little you masturbate when you're young won't have anything to do with what type of orgasms are most intense for you when you're an adult.

Is masturbation "sinful" or morally wrong?
One person's idea of what's "sinful" or morally wrong may be quite different from another person's. Nowadays, most people do not think masturbation is morally wrong or sinful, and personally, we go along with that point of view. In the past, many religions held that masturbation was a sin, and although many religious leaders no longer feel this way, some still do. The Cath-

olic religion's official point of view holds that masturbation is a sin. This doesn't mean, however, that all Catholics or even all Catholic priests and church leaders feel this way.

People who consider masturbation a sin often point to the story of Onan in the Bible (Genesis, Chapter 3, verses 9-10), in which Onan is punished by God for "spilling his seed on the ground." They feel that the story of Onan is a story about masturbation (masturbation used to be called onanism), and that it shows that God disapproves of masturbation. Others don't feel that this is what the story of Onan is all about. People who think masturbation is sinful usually feel that God approves of a man ejaculating only during intercourse with his wife, and that a man should practice enough self-control so that he only ejaculates under those circumstances.

As we said, what one person thinks is sinful or morally wrong may be different from what another person thinks. It's an individual thing, something you'll have to decide for yourself. If you're bothered by the notion that masturbation may be sinful or morally wrong, perhaps you should talk with your minister, priest, or religious leader, or maybe you'll find some of the publications we've listed in the back of this book helpful.

Is it weird for a boy to masturbate with other boys?
Some boys have their first experience with masturbation by watching other boys, and it's not unusual for groups of boys to masturbate together. Some boys also experiment with masturbation by touching another boy's penis, by masturbating another boy to the point of orgasm, or by letting another boy masturbate them. Boys who do this often worry about whether this is

weird. Sometimes they think that this means that they are homosexual.

Homosexuals are people who prefer to have sexual contacts with people who are the same sex as they are. Most adults in our society are *heterosexuals*, which means that they prefer to have sexual experiences with people of the opposite sex. We'll talk more about homosexuality in Chapter 9, but for now you should know that masturbating with other boys, masturbating another boy, or thinking about doing either of these things does not mean you are a homosexual. Many boys engage in some form of what we call "sex play" with other boys as they're growing up, just as some girls engage in sex play with other girls, and some kids engage in sex play with members of the opposite sex as they're growing up. None of these sexual experiences is at all weird in the sense of being uncommon or unusual. If you've had such experiences and have wondered about them or felt uncomfortable, be sure to read Chapter 9, where we talk more about these things.

Do married people masturbate?

Yes, many people masturbate even though they have regular sex partners. They may masturbate privately (that is, when they're alone), or they may include masturbation as part of their sex lives with each other. They may masturbate before they have intercourse as a way of "warming up" or getting ready. Or they may masturbate instead of having intercourse, especially if the couple doesn't want to take the risk of the woman getting pregnant. (Unless a man ejaculates in the vagina or near the opening of the vagina, the sperm can't get

homosexual (hoe-moe-SEK-shoo-well)
heterosexual (HET-er-oh-SEK-shoo-well)
homosexuality (hoe-moe-sek-shoo-WAL-ity)

into her uterus and tubes to fertilize the ovum.) If a man ejaculates before the woman has an orgasm, masturbation can be a way for her to have an orgasm even though his penis is no longer erect and they can't continue having intercourse.

If a boy doesn't masturbate or have sexual intercourse, what happens to all the sperm?
If a boy doesn't ejaculate, either through masturbation or intercourse, one of two things may happen. As the ampulla becomes full, the sperm may simply dribble into the urethra, be mixed in with his urine, and be eliminated from his body when he urinates. Or he may have a wet dream.

WET DREAMS

As we explained earlier in this chapter, boys sometimes ejaculate while they're asleep. A common term for this is "having a wet dream." The scientific name for wet dreams is nocturnal emissions. *Nocturnal* means "during the night," and *emissions* are things that are "emitted" or "sent forth." So nocturnal emissions are ejaculations (sperm emitted or sent forth) at night.

It's possible for a grown man to have a wet dream, but they are much more common among boys going through puberty. Not all boys have wet dreams at this time in their lives, but many do. A boy who masturbates regularly is less likely to have a wet dream than one who never or only rarely masturbates. However, even boys who masturbate may have wet dreams fairly often.

Many boys have their first ejaculation during a wet dream. If you don't know about wet dreams and haven't

nocturnal (nok-TUR-nul)
emissions (e-MISH-uns)

been prepared for the fact that it may happen to you, a wet dream can be a confusing experience. Many boys thought they'd wet their beds or were bleeding or something until they realized that the fluid was milky white, not like blood or urine. As one man we interviewed explained:

I'm what?—sixty-seven years old—so this is over fifty years ago, but I still remember my first wet dream like it was yesterday. Nobody told me anything about anything. So I woke up in the middle of the night. There's this wet, sticky stuff all over my belly. I thought, jeez, I wet my bed—at my age! I was thirteen or fourteen at the time.

So a few days, maybe a week later, it happens again. Only now I pay more attention, and it's not piss [urine]. It's white and thick like a lotion or cream, sticky. I think I've got some kind of sickness. It keeps happening, so finally I tell my mother. She says if I control myself and don't think about "such things," it won't happen. I have no idea what she's talking about—control myself from what? Don't think about what things? I wasn't thinking about anything. I was asleep.

Charlie, age 67

Even if you know about wet dreams beforehand, they can be a surprising experience, as one boy told me after class one day:

My mom and dad had told me all about this kind of stuff ever since I was a kid. Still, it was a surprise the first time. Everything was hazy, but there was this wetness on my pajamas, and for a while I couldn't figure things out. I was only half awake. Then as I woke up more, I thought, "Oh, yeah, this is what Mom had said about."

Regardless of whether or not you know about wet dreams beforehand, you may feel embarrassed if you have one. One of the films I use in my sex-education classes, a film called *Am I Normal?*, deals with one young boy's experience as he's going through puberty. In one scene, the boy wakes up after having had a wet dream. He's so embarrassed that he takes off his pajamas and the sheets off his bed and sneaks down the hall to the bathroom. He turns the water on in the sink and pours a glass of water over his bedclothes and stuffs them in the laundry hamper. His mom hears him and calls out, "Is that you, honey? Is there anything wrong?"

"Nothing, Mom. . . . Oh, by the way, Mom, I forgot to tell you . . . I spilled water all over my bed," he nervously explains. "I guess I'm going to have to put my sheets in the hamper."

The boys in my class always get a big laugh out of this scene, probably because many of them have felt the same kind of embarrassment. But wet dreams aren't anything to be embarrassed about. They're a natural and normal thing, just another part of growing up.

After the class in which I show this film, there are usually at least a couple of questions about wet dreams in the Everything You Ever Wanted to Know question box. Two questions that come up over and over again are, "Do wet dreams only happen at night?" and "Do they only happen when you're asleep?" The answer is that wet dreams could happen anytime you're asleep. If you took a nap during the day, it would be possible for you to have a wet dream. But wet dreams only happen when you're asleep. You don't ejaculate when you're awake unless you decide to ejaculate. You might have a spontaneous erection, an erection that happens all by itself, but you won't have an ejaculation unless you deliberately engage in some form of sexual stimulation, such as masturbation.

The kids in my class also want to know why they're called *wet dreams*. "Do they only happen if you're having a dream?" "Do you have to be having a sexy dream?" they ask. The fact of the matter is that everyone dreams when he or she is asleep. Even if you don't remember doing so, you've been having dreams (a fact scientists have discovered by studying the electrical patterns in the brains of sleeping people). But the term *wet dream* doesn't mean that you dream during a nocturnal emission. It just refers to the fact that wet dreams happen when you're asleep, or at least half asleep. You may have been having a "sexy dream" during your nocturnal emission. Many boys who awake to find that they have ejaculated recall that their dream was about something sexual. But you may have a wet dream even if you haven't been having a sexual dream.

By the way, Charlie's mother was wrong. A boy can't stop himself from having wet dreams. They're just something that happens. They're completely natural and normal, and, like masturbation, are part of your body's way of emptying out the ampulla and making way for new sperm.

After you've read this far in the book, you've probably learned just about everything you've ever wanted to know about what happens to a boy's body during puberty. But we haven't talked very much about what happens to *girls'* bodies. So in the next chapter, we'll learn about girls and puberty.

CHAPTER 6

Girls and Puberty

Each year my daughter, Area, and I get together with a bunch of our friends and rent a houseboat. We spend a week cruising up and down the California Delta, the series of rivers that lead into the San Francisco Bay. We swim and fish and dig for clams and have mud fights and lie around in the sun and have a wonderful time just doing nothing at all. It's pretty much the same group of us every year. All of the adults are single mothers or single fathers, and we all have daughters about the same age. The girls went to grade school together. In fact, that's how we adults got to know one another in the first place.

We've been getting together like this for a number of years. Our daughters are teenagers now, and they go to different schools. Even though we've all gone our separate ways since the girls were little—some of us have even moved to different cities or towns—we still get together every year for this houseboat cruise.

Well, one year it just so happened that Area and I were putting the finishing touches on the book about girls and puberty when it came time for our annual cruise. Because we were going to spend a week on board a boat with six teenage girls, I figured that I'd take the rough draft of the book along and try to talk the girls into reading through the various chapters and making comments or suggestions. The girls were all about the same age, but they were in various stages of puberty. I thought that the more developed ones might be interested in the later chapters and that the girls who weren't so developed might want to read the earlier chapters.

I was wrong. All the girls wanted to read the same chapter—the one about boys. They couldn't have cared less about the rest of the book! They grabbed that chapter and went giggling off to the roof of the houseboat with their towels and suntan lotion and read it together. Later on, some of the girls read other chapters, but the big hit was definitely the chapter about boys.

I think their reaction was a pretty normal one. As we're going through puberty, we usually get at least some information about what's happening to our own bodies, if not from our parents and teachers, then from our friends. A lot of times, though, parents and teachers don't tell us about what's happening to the opposite sex. (They may feel that we just don't need to know this information, or that telling us will make us "too interested" in the opposite sex or will make us want to rush out and have sexual intercourse.) Our friends may not know much more about this subject than we do.

All this makes it difficult for us to find out what's going on, and not knowing how puberty happens in the opposite sex can make everything seem a lot more confusing and mysterious than it needs to be. So in this

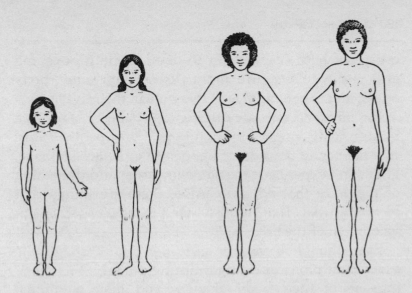

Illustration 22. Puberty in girls. As a girl goes through puberty, her hips get wider. Fat tissue begins to grow around her hips, thighs, and buttocks, giving her body a curvier shape. Her breasts begin to swell, and soft nests of hair begin to grow under her arms and on her genitals.

chapter, we'll be talking about how puberty happens in girls' bodies. If you're like most boys, you'll probably be pretty curious about this. (In fact, we wouldn't be surprised if this was the first chapter you turned to in this book.)

SIMILARITIES AND DIFFERENCES

As you can see from Illustration 22, girls' bodies also change quite a bit as they go through puberty. In some ways, puberty in girls is similar to puberty in boys. Both sexes undergo a growth spurt and a change in the general shape of their body. Both boys and girls begin to grow pubic hair. Boys start to make sperm for the first time, and girls produce their first ripe ova. The genital organs of both sexes begin to develop. Both boys and girls begin to perspire more, to take on adult body odors, and to get pimples at this time in their lives.

But boys and girls are different, so puberty happens a bit differently in girls than in boys. Some of the things that happen to boys don't happen to girls. For instance, girls don't experience the same lowering and deepening of the voice that boys do. Also, there are things that happen to girls that don't happen to boys, such as development of the breasts.

Even though boys and girls don't go through the exact same physical changes during puberty, their feelings about their body changes and their emotional reactions to growing up are, as we shall see, very similar. Let's start with the physical changes.

THE GROWTH SPURT

Like boys, girls go through a growth spurt during puberty and start to grow taller at a faster rate. The girls' growth spurt usually happens about two years before the boys' growth spurt. So at the age of eleven or twelve, girls often grow taller than the boys their age. However, a couple of years later, when the boys begin their growth spurt, they start to catch up to the girls. The boys' growth spurt lasts longer than the girls', and boys tend to add more inches during this time, so boys usually end up being taller than girls. Of course, there are some girls who will always be taller than most of the boys. But often a girl who is taller than the boys in her class when she's eleven or twelve will find that the boys have caught up by the age of thirteen or fourteen.

CHANGING SHAPE

The general shape, or contour, of a girl's body also changes as she goes through puberty. Her hips get wider, and fat tissue grows around the hips, buttocks, and thighs. This gives her body a curvier, rounder, more "womanly" shape.

PUBIC HAIR

Girls, too, begin to grow hair during puberty. In girls, the pubic hair begins to grow on the vulva. For some girls, this is the first change they notice as they begin puberty.

Just as doctors have divided the growth of the male sex organs into five stages, so they've divided the development of female pubic hair into five stages, shown in Illustration 23. Stage 1 is the childhood stage. It begins at birth and continues until a girl reaches Stage 2. A girl doesn't have any pubic hair during Stage 1. Stage 2 starts when the first curly pubic hairs appear, which is generally around the age of eleven, although it can happen earlier or later.

During Stage 3, the pubic hairs get darker and curlier. There are more of them, and they cover a wider area. Girls usually reach Stage 3 around the age of twelve. In Stage 4, which usually occurs between the ages of twelve and thirteen, the pubic hair gets still thicker and curlier and covers an even wider area.

Stage 5 is the adult stage. The pubic hair grows in an upside-down triangle pattern. In some women, the pubic hair grows up toward the belly button or out toward the thighs. The typical girl reaches this stage around the age of fourteen.

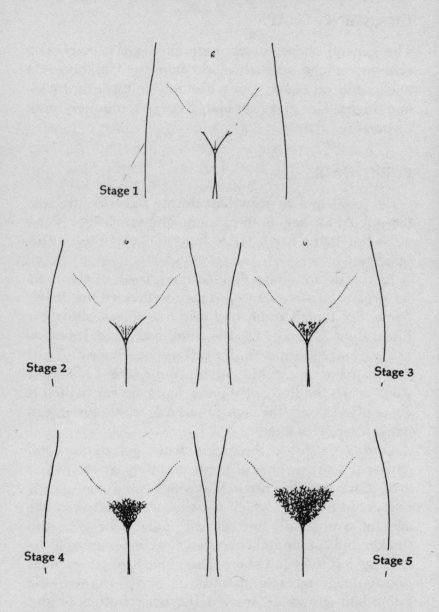

Illustration 23. The five stages of a girl's pubic hair growth

BREASTS

You may have heard all sorts of slang words used to refer to a girl's breasts—"boobs," "boobies," "knockers," "melons," "jugs," "tits," "titties," or whatever. Regardless of what you call them, you've probably noticed that they grow larger during puberty. Doctors have divided female breast development into the five stages shown in Illustration 24.

Stage 1 is the childhood stage. The breasts have not yet begun to develop. Stage 2 is the beginning of breast development. A small, buttonlike mound, similar to the ones some boys develop, forms under each nipple. The breasts may be sore or tender or even downright painful, especially if they're hit. The nipple gets larger, and the areola gets wider. Both the nipple and areola get darker in color, and the buttonlike mound underneath causes them to swell and stand out from the chest more. Most girls reach Stage 2 around the age of eleven.

In Stages 3 and 4, the breasts continue to get larger, rounder, and fuller, and they stand out from the chest more. The average girl reaches Stage 3 when she's about twelve, and Stage 4 when she's about thirteen. Girls stay in Stage 4 of breast development for a while, and most don't reach Stage 5 until they are about fifteen. Of course, not all girls are average, so some will reach these stages when they're a bit younger, and some when they're a bit older. Stage 5 is the adult stage.

Just as the age at which a boy starts to go through the various stages of puberty doesn't have anything to do with how quickly he goes through those stages, so the age at which a girl starts to go through pubic hair and breast development doesn't have anything to do with how quickly she gets to the adult stage. Some early starters develop quickly and some slowly; the same

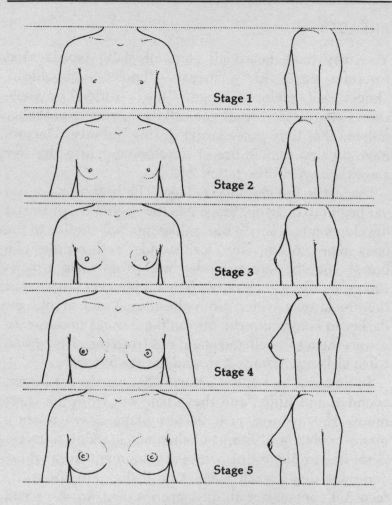

Illustration 24. The five stages of breast development

thing happens with late starters. There are some girls who develop *very* quickly. Such girls may start Stage 2 and reach Stage 3 within six months. After another six months, they've reached Stage 5. Other girls take six or more years to go from Stage 2 to Stage 5. The typical girl takes about four years to go from Stage 2 to Stage 5.

The stages of pubic hair growth and breast development may go together, so that a girl is in, say, Stage 3 of breast development at the same time that she's in Stage 3 of pubic hair development. However, these stages don't always coincide. For example, a girl might be in Stage 3 of breast development but only Stage 2 of pubic hair growth. Or she might be in Stage 4 of breast development but only Stage 2 of pubic hair growth.

You may be curious as to why a girl's breasts start to grow larger. Like the other changes that happen during puberty, this one occurs because the girl's body is getting ready for a time in her life when she may decide to have children. In order to understand why a girl's breasts grow, you have to know what's happening inside her breasts. Illustration 25 shows the inside of a grown woman's breast. Each breast is made up of fifteen to twenty-five separate compartments called *lobes*, although you can see only three of them in this picture. The lobes are packed together like separate sections of an orange. They are surrounded by a cushion of fat tissue. Inside each lobe is a treelike structure. The leaves of this tree are the *alveoli*. When a woman has a baby, milk is made inside these leaves. The milk travels from the leaves, through the branches and trunks of the tree (which are called milk ducts), to the nipple. When a mother breast-feeds, the baby sucks on the nipple and milk comes out.

As a girl begins puberty, she starts to develop milk ducts, alveoli, and fat tissue to cushion these milk-producing organs. Her breasts aren't yet ready to make milk and won't be until after she has had a baby. But

alveoli (al-VEE-oh-lie)

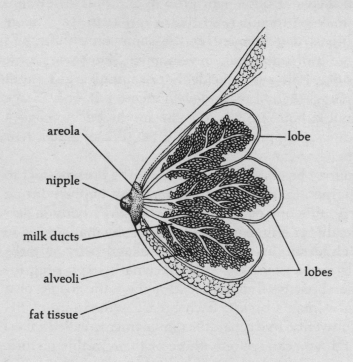

areola

nipple

milk ducts

alveoli

fat tissue

lobe

lobes

Illustration 25. Cross section of a woman's breast

her body is getting ready for this possibility, which is why her breasts grow larger.

Feelings about Developing Breasts

Just as some boys worry about whether their penis is "big enough," so girls often worry about the size of their breasts. Many girls (and women, too) wish their breasts were larger. Women with large breasts are supposed to be more feminine, more womanly, or sexier than smaller-breasted women. At least, that's the idea that you might get from all the big-breasted, glamorous women we see in advertisements, on TV, and in movies.

But the size of a woman's breasts doesn't have anything to do with how feminine or sexual she is, no more than the size of a man's penis has anything to do with how masculine or sexually powerful he is. Like a penis, breasts work equally well (produce the same amount of milk) regardless of their size.

Bras

As their breasts are developing, many girls begin to wear bras. Some wear them so that their breasts don't jiggle around when they run or dance or play sports, which can be uncomfortable. The support the bra gives makes them feel more comfortable. Some girls wear bras because they feel self-conscious without them. Others don't wear bras at all. It's an individual thing, a matter of personal choice.

BODY HAIR, PERSPIRATION, PIMPLES, AND OTHER CHANGES

Girls also grow new hair on their arms and legs during puberty, although such body hair isn't usually as thick as it is on boys. Some girls shave the hair on their legs with razors or use chemical hair removers to get rid of the hair. Others don't bother. Again, this is an individual thing, a matter of personal choice.

Underarm hair also develops during puberty, and some girls shave this hair. Perspiration and oil glands in the genital area, the underarms, the face, neck, shoulders, and back also become more active in girls during puberty, just as they do in boys. Some girls choose to use underarm deodorants; others don't. Some women use the deodorant sprays made for the vulvar and vaginal area. But these sprays can cause irritations, so we don't think they're a good idea.

Beginning with puberty, a girl's genitals may have a moister feeling due to the change in the oil and sweat glands in this area.

Pimples, acne, and stretch marks may be a problem for girls, just as they are for some boys.

THE GENITALS

A boy's scrotum and penis develop and change during puberty, and a girl's genital organs also change in appearance. Pubic hair grows on the mons and outer lips. The mons, the outer lips, and the inner lips get fatter and fleshier. The lips get larger, more wrinkly, and darker in color. The clitoris, urinary opening, and vaginal opening get a bit larger too.

The Hymen

A girl's *hymen* also gets thicker and more noticeable during puberty. The hymen is a thin piece of skin tissue that lies just inside the vaginal opening. Slang terms for it are "cherry" or "maidenhead."

The hymen looks different in different women. In some, it may be just a thin fringe of skin around the edges of the opening to the vagina. It may stretch across the opening and have one or more holes in it. Illustration 26 shows a close-up of different women's vaginal openings and some of the ways a hymen may look.

In young girls, the hymen may not be very noticeable. During puberty, it usually gets thicker, more rigid, and more noticeable. Not every female has a noticeable hymen, though. A few women are simply born without one. Other women's hymens are so small and thin that it's hard to see them.

hymen (HI-men)

As strange as it seems, this tiny piece of skin was once considered *very* important by many people. People used to think that all women had the kind of hymen that stretches all the way across the vaginal opening. They thought that the only way a hymen could be stretched or torn was if a man put his penis inside a woman's vagina while they were having sex. Today, we know this isn't true. For one thing, a few females simply don't have hymens. Of those that do, not all have the kind that stretches all the way across the vaginal opening. Some have a hymen that is just a fringe of tissue around the edges of the vaginal opening; some have such a small, thin one that it's hard to see. Also, hymens can get stretched or torn in a number of ways. Horseback riding, doing a split, falling off a bike, or a stretching movement can tear the hymen, though this is not common. Whether or not a woman has a hymen doesn't necessarily have anything to do with whether or not she has had sex with a man. In fact, some women have sexual intercourse quite a number of times without their hymen stretching or tearing at all.

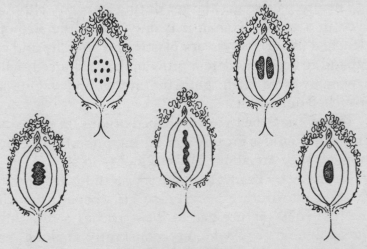

Illustration 26. Hymens

When the hymen is stretched or torn—whether it's during sex or while a girl is doing gymnastics or riding a horse or whatever—it may bleed a little, somewhat, or not at all. It may hurt a little, somewhat, or not at all. But only rarely does a hymen bleed or hurt so badly that a doctor's care is needed. In fact, most girls and women never have any problems at all.

THE VAGINA, UTERUS, AND OVARIES

Another change that happens in a girl's body during puberty is that the sex organs on the inside of her body begin to develop and grow. (Turn back to Illustration 6, page 20, to see these organs again.) The vagina gets longer, until it reaches its adult length of three to five inches. This still isn't very large, and as you may recall, the average penis is about six inches long when it's erect. But the vagina is very elastic and stretchy, so the penis can easily fit inside when a man and a woman are having sexual intercourse.

The uterus also gets larger during puberty, although even in a grown woman it is only about the size of a clenched fist. It, too, is very elastic and stretchy and can expand to accommodate a growing baby. Indeed, when a woman gives birth, both the uterus and vagina are stretched quite a bit.

The ovaries, the two egg-shaped organs on either side of the uterus, also grow larger during puberty. In grown women, they are about 1½ to 2 inches in size.

Just as a boy begins to make sperm in his testicles for the first time during puberty, so girls begin producing the first fully mature ova in their ovaries at this time. But unlike males, who are constantly making new sperm in their bodies, females have all the ova they'll ever have when they're born. They don't make new ova every day. The ova they have when they're born are not fully mature or ripe, however. The first ovum doesn't fully ripen and leave the ovary until after a girl has already started puberty and begun to develop pubic hair and breasts.

During puberty, a girl *ovulates* for the first time. A ripe ovum leaves her ovary; in fact, it pops right off. This process of popping a ripe ovum off the ovary is called *ovulation*. As soon as the ovum pops off, the fringed ends of the fallopian tubes reach out like tiny fingers to grasp the ovum and pull it into the tube. (see Illustration 27). The fallopian tubes are very tiny, no bigger around than a strand of spaghetti and only about four inches long. The inside of each tube is lined with tiny hairs, which are connected to the muscles in the walls of the tubes. The muscles contract and loosen up rhythmically. This causes the tiny hairs to sway back and forth and to sweep the ovum along the length of the tube toward the uterus.

If a girl has sexual intercourse at just about the time she releases her first ripe ovum, and if the male has ejaculated sperm into her vagina, it's possible that one of his sperm could swim through her uterus, into her tubes, and meet up with and fertilize her first ripe ovum. But this doesn't usually happen. For one thing, most girls ovulate and produce their first ripe ovum when they're only about thirteen, and most girls of this age don't have sexual intercourse.

Even if a girl *did* have sexual intercourse just around the time that she released her first ovum from her ovary,

ovulates (AHV-u-lates)
ovulation (ahv-u-LAY-shun)

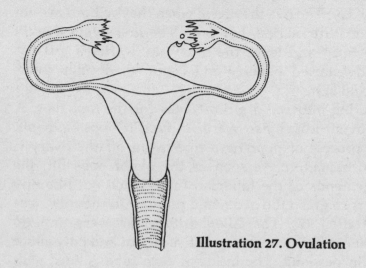

Illustration 27. Ovulation

and a sperm met up with it in the fallopian tube, the ovum probably wouldn't be fertilized by the sperm. The first ovum isn't really a fully mature one. It's sort of a "practice" ovum. It's *possible* for one of these "practice" ova to be fertilized, but it's very unusual. Usually, then, a girl's first ovum travels to the uterus without being fertilized. After a few days of floating around inside the uterus, the ovum simply disintegrates.

HORMONES

Like boys, girls begin to make new hormones in their bodies during puberty. As you may recall from reading Chapter 4, there's a gland in a boy's brain called the pituitary gland, and a few years before puberty it starts to make small amounts of certain hormones. These hormones travel to a boy's testicles and cause them to start making a hormone of their own called testosterone. At first, neither his pituitary nor his testicles make very much hormone, but as he grows older, a boy makes increasing amounts of pituitary hormones in his brain. This, in turn, causes his testicles to make more and more testosterone. The testosterone travels to other parts of his body and causes changes such as the enlargement of his penis and scrotum, the growth of pubic, facial, and body hair, and the lowering of his voice.

Girls, too, have pituitary glands in their brains. A few years before puberty begins, a girl's pituitary gland starts making the same hormones that a boy's pituitary makes. In girls, though, these pituitary hormones travel to the ovaries. Like the testicles, the ovaries are also glands and are also capable of making hormones. One of the hormones that a girl's ovaries make is called *estrogen*.

As she grows older, a girl's brain makes increasing amounts of pituitary hormone. This, in turn, causes her ovaries to make increasing amounts of estrogen. Just as testosterone from a boy's testicles travels to other parts of his body and causes puberty changes like pubic hair and the growth of his penis, so estrogen from a girl's ovaries travels to other parts of her body and causes certain puberty changes. For instance, estrogen is responsible for the growth of her pubic hair and the development of her breasts.

Estrogen also causes changes on the inside of a girl's uterus. The uterus is a hollow organ. The inside walls of the uterus are covered by a special lining. Before puberty, this lining is very thin. Once puberty starts and a girl is making increasing amounts of estrogen, this lining begins to grow thicker. It becomes very spongy and soft and fills with blood. By the time a girl has begun her growth spurt, sprouted pubic hair, and de-

estrogen (ES-tro-jen)

veloped breasts, the lining of her uterus has grown quite thick.

Like the other changes that happen during puberty, this takes place because a girl's body is getting ready for a time in her life when she may decide to have a baby. When and if she does become pregnant, this lining is very important. After her ovum is fertilized by a sperm in the fallopian tube, it will travel to the uterus and plant itself in the thick lining there. The lining will provide the blood and nutrients a fertilized ovum needs in order to grow into a baby.

THE MENSTRUAL PERIOD

As we've explained, a girl's first ovum isn't fertilized by a sperm. It doesn't plant itself in the uterine lining; instead, it simply disintegrates. Because the ovum hasn't been fertilized, there's no longer any need for the thick lining that has grown on the inside walls of the uterus, so the uterus begins to shed the lining. The tissues of the bloody lining begin to break up and turn very liquidy. The bloody and liquidy tissue collect at the bottom of the uterus. They dribble out the opening in the bottom of the uterus that leads to the vagina. Then the blood and liquid flow down the vaginal walls and dribble out the vaginal opening (see Illustration 28).

When a girl begins bleeding from her vaginal opening, we say she is *menstruating* or having her *menstrual period*. A girl generally has her first menstrual period sometime between the ages of nine and sixteen. The average age is about thirteen.

It takes about three to seven days for the uterus to

menstruating (MEN-stroo-ate-ing)
menstrual (MEN-strool)

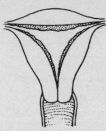

As the ovum is ripening in the ovary, the lining of the uterus gets thicker

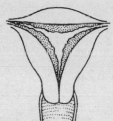

and thicker.

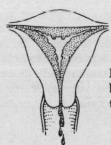

If the ovum is not fertilized, the lining begins to break down and dribble out of the body through the vagina.

Illustration 28. Cross section of the uterus. The shaded area is the lining of the uterus. It breaks down and is shed during menstruation.

completely shed the lining. Altogether, about half a cup of blood comes out of the girl's vagina during her menstrual period. While she's bleeding like this, a girl usually wears a pad of cotton, called a sanitary pad or napkin, inside her underpants to catch the blood. Or she may insert a cotton plug, called a tampon, into her vagina to absorb the blood (see Illustration 29). She changes this pad or tampon several times a day.

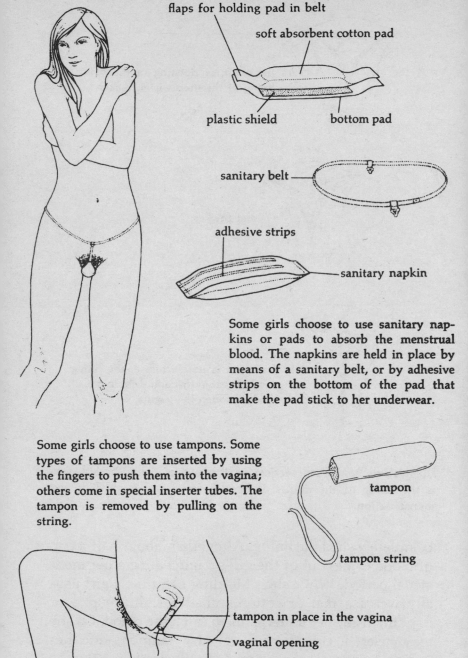

flaps for holding pad in belt

soft absorbent cotton pad

plastic shield   bottom pad

sanitary belt

adhesive strips

sanitary napkin

Some girls choose to use sanitary napkins or pads to absorb the menstrual blood. The napkins are held in place by means of a sanitary belt, or by adhesive strips on the bottom of the pad that make the pad stick to her underwear.

Some girls choose to use tampons. Some types of tampons are inserted by using the fingers to push them into the vagina; others come in special inserter tubes. The tampon is removed by pulling on the string.

tampon

tampon string

tampon in place in the vagina

vaginal opening

Illustration 29. Sanitary napkins and tampon

The Menstrual Cycle

After the uterus has completely shed the lining and the girl stops bleeding, the lining starts to grow thick and spongy again. While this is happening, the ovaries are getting ready to ovulate again. Around nine or ten days after a girl finishes her menstrual bleeding, another ovum pops off one of her ovaries. It, too, travels through the fallopian tube toward the uterus. Unless it is fertilized by a sperm in the tube, it won't plant in the uterine lining either and will once again disintegrate.

Because the ovum hasn't been fertilized, the newly grown lining isn't needed. So it breaks down and dribbles out of the uterus into the vagina, and the process starts up again:

- The girl starts bleeding.
- The bleeding lasts for a few days or maybe a week or so, and then it stops.
- The lining of the uterus starts to grow thick and spongy again.
- The ovary releases another ripe ovum.
- The fingerlike ends of the fallopian tube grasp the ovum and pull it into the tube.
- The hairs inside the tube sweep the ovum toward the uterus.
- Unless the ovum is fertilized, it disintegrates inside the uterus.
- The newly grown lining breaks down and dribbles down the vaginal walls and out the vaginal opening.
- The girl starts bleeding and having another menstrual period.

The whole process, which is called the menstrual cycle, takes about a month. The cycle repeats itself, month after month, over and over again, year in and year out, throughout most of a woman's life. Once she gets to be about forty-five to fifty-five years old, the cycle stops. The woman stops ovulating and menstruating each month. This stopping of the monthly cycle is called *menopause*.

Between puberty, the time when she first starts menstruating, and menopause, the time when she stops menstruating, a female generally has her period pretty regularly, about once a month. This isn't a hard and fast rule, though. There are lots of exceptions. For one thing, women stop menstruating when they get pregnant. If a sperm fertilizes an ovum in the fallopian tube, the fertilized ovum travels to the uterus and plants itself in the uterine lining. The lining provides the blood and nourishment the fertilized ovum needs to grow into a baby. So for the nine months of her pregnancy, while the baby is growing inside her uterus, a woman doesn't shed her uterine lining. (Here again, there are exceptions to the rule; occasionally, a woman will have one or even two periods after she's gotten pregnant. But such periods are shorter than normal periods, and most women don't have their periods at all once the ovum has been fertilized.) After childbirth, the woman's periods may start up again within a few weeks or a month or two, or it may take several months before they start again.

Also, young girls who've just started menstruating don't always have their periods regularly, once a month. It usually takes a while for the body to adjust to menstruating. Many girls have their first period and then don't have a second one for a number of months. Some have their second period just a couple of weeks after their first. Girls often don't start having their periods very regularly until they've been menstruating for two or three years.

menopause (MEN-o-pause)

There are certain medical problems that can cause a woman to miss one or more menstrual periods or to stop menstruating altogether. Even healthy women without a single medical problem sometimes miss a period or two. Gaining or losing a lot of weight, moving to a new home, traveling, stress, excitement, nervousness, emotional ups and downs—all these can cause a female to miss her period. And there are some perfectly healthy females who only menstruate a few times a year. That's just the way their particular bodies work.

Most of the time, though, *most* women have their menstrual periods pretty regularly, about once a month. By "pretty regularly," we don't mean that it happens once every thirty days exactly. There's a lot of variation. Some women have periods that come as close together as every twenty-one days; others have periods that come as far apart as every thirty-six days. The average is about twenty-eight days.

No woman's period is like clockwork. One month the menstrual cycle may last twenty-five days; the next month it may last twenty-eight days; and the following month, thirty days. One month the bleeding may last for three days, the next month for five days. Some women's periods vary quite a bit, and others are more regular. In general, though, a woman's period comes about once a month and lasts for a few days to a week or so.

The First Period
Some girls are excited about the prospect of having their periods; others aren't so eager. Many girls are concerned that their first period will sneak up on them. They worry that the blood will soak through their

clothes without their realizing it and they'll be publicly embarrassed. Such things can happen, but generally a girl has a sensation of wetness and has plenty of time to get to the bathroom before the blood soaks through her underclothes. Besides, not that much blood comes out all at once. Altogether over the entire period, only about half a cup to a cup of blood is lost, so only a small amount is dribbling out of the vaginal opening at any one time.

Most girls use sanitary napkins or pads instead of tampons at first. A lot of girls think that a virgin, a girl who hasn't had sex yet, can't use a tampon because of the hymen. But as we explained, the hymen has openings in it and is very stretchy. Unless a girl has a particularly rigid or tight hymen, she can use a tampon regardless of whether or not she's had sexual intercourse. Still, most girls prefer to use napkins at first, unless they want to go swimming, in which case they use a tampon.

Menstrual Cramps

Menstrual cramps are abdominal pains that may occur early in the menstrual period or a few days before the period actually starts. Cramps may vary from a feeling of fullness or pressure, to a dull, achy feeling, to a sharp pain or spasm. Almost every woman has cramps at some time in her life, but for most they're not a real problem and don't interfere with their daily activities. There are, however, some women who have such severe cramps that they actually have to spend a few days in bed each month.

Severe cramps can be a sign of some underlying medical problem, and women who have severe cramps should see a doctor. Often, though, the doctor is unable to pinpoint a cause for the cramps. Many doctors used to think that cramps were "all in your head," and some doctors still think this. Recently, though, medical research has shown that women who have cramps often have unusually high levels of hormones called *prostaglandins*, which cause the uterus to contract painfully during menstruation. There are now anti-prostaglandin medications available to help such women. For most women, though, their cramps, if they have them at all, aren't uncomfortable enough for them to need medication. If they do need to take something, aspirin will usually do the trick.

Other Menstrual Changes

Some women notice other physical or emotional changes at certain points in their menstrual cycle. For example, I get very energetic during my period and often get into fits of housecleaning (which is nice because, most of the time, I'm not too enthusiastic about housework). About a week and a half before my period starts, my breasts swell a bit and get very tender, or sometimes downright painful. (This started happening only after I turned thirty.) For a couple of years after I turned thirty-two, I started having moderate cramps during the first couple of days of my period. I'd never had them before, and lately they seem to have disappeared again. I always know when I'm going to ovulate because I get to feeling very sexual.

Some girls and women don't notice any changes associated with their menstrual cycles; others do. Sometimes these changes are pleasant ones—extra energy, an especially "up" or good feeling, bursts of creativity. Sometimes they're negative—tension, irritability, head-

prostaglandins (pros-ta-GLAN-dins)

aches, bowel problems, swelling, and temporary weight gain. Some women notice that they're cranky right before their period starts, or that they are more apt to get depressed at this time. Some notice a slight twinge or cramps for a day or so about two weeks before their period starts. This is about when ovulation occurs, so this pain is sometimes called ovulation pain. For most women, though, the ovum pops off the ovary without their really noticing it.

Myths about Menstruation

People used to believe all sorts of crazy things about menstruation. Primitive tribes used to think that you'd get sick if you ate food cooked by a menstruating woman, that her glance could wither a field of crops, that having sex with a menstruating woman could make a man's penis fall off. Some tribes even banished women to menstrual huts each month during their period. Some of the slang terms used for menstruation—"the curse," "falling off the roof," "on the rag"—reflect these old, negative attitudes toward menstruation.

Today, we know that none of these things is true. A woman can have sex while she's menstruating and no harm will come to her sex partner. In fact, a menstruating woman can do anything during her period that she'd do at any other time. Old notions have a way of hanging on, though, and there are still some people who think that a menstruating woman shouldn't have sex, take a bath, wash her hair, drink cold drinks, or exercise, and that doing these things will cause a heavier flow, make her period last longer, or give her cramps. None of these things is true. In fact, sexual intercourse and exercise are often helpful for women who are troubled by cramps.

In the first six chapters of this book, we've tried to answer the questions you may have had about how puberty happens. But there may still be other questions you'd like answered. In Chapters 7 and 9 we will talk about a number of other topics related to puberty and sexuality, and you may find the answers to your questions there.

CHAPTER 7

Sexual Intercourse, Pregnancy and Childbirth, and Birth Control

The changes that take place in boys' and girls' bodies during puberty happen because their bodies are getting ready for a time in their lives when they may want to reproduce—that is, make a baby. Many of the kids in my classes have matured to the point where they're making sperm or ovulating and are physically capable of reproduction. But they aren't ready to become parents yet, not by a long shot! In fact, if you're like most of the boys and girls in my classes, you probably spend about as much time thinking about having babies as you do thinking how you could help out around the house by doing more chores or what you'd pack to take on a trip to the moon.

Even though the kids in my class aren't planning to have babies any time soon, they're still curious about how babies are made, so we spend a fair amount of

reproduce (REE-preh-DOOSE)
reproduction (REE-preh-DUCK-shun)

time in class talking about reproduction and things like sexual intercourse, pregnancy, and childbirth. I even show a videotape which shows a baby being born, and although the kids always say it's the "most totally gross thing ever," I notice that they keep begging me to show this tape year after year.

Once we've talked about intercourse, pregnancy, and childbirth in class, the kids' questions usually lead us around to another topic—ways of preventing pregnancy. So we also spend a fair amount of time talking about birth control, especially in my classes for older kids. In this chapter, we're going to be talking about these topics in pretty much the same order as we talk about them in class.

My students have about ten zillion questions on these topics. There simply isn't room in just this one chapter to answer all of them, but we'll try to answer the most commonly asked ones, and hopefully, you'll find answers to some of your questions here. If you find that some sections of this chapter are too complicated or simply don't interest you, ask for help from your parent, or skip it altogether.

SEXUAL INTERCOURSE
The boys and girls in my classes and the kids who write to us are *very* curious about this topic. We explained a bit about sexual intercourse way back in Chapter 1, on page 9 and pages 15–18, and also in Chapter 5 on pages 104–105. You may want to take another look at those pages before you read the questions and answers in this section.

I don't quite understand how the penis fits into the vagina when a man and woman have sex. Could you explain or show us a picture?
There's an old saying, "A picture is worth a thousand words," and we agree. So, we've included Illustration

30 here, which shows an erect penis fitting into the vagina in just one of the many positions a couple may use for intercourse.

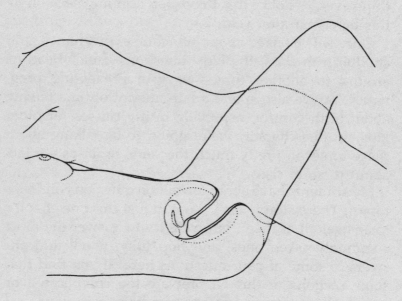

Illustration 30. Penis in vagina

What's the first thing you should do when you have sex? Could you explain to us, step by step, what people do when they're having sex?
Sexual intercourse isn't something that has specific rules you have to follow. When children go out to the playground after school, they don't have a specific set of directions. No one tells them that first they must take five steps, then do three somersaults, then swing on the swing for five minutes, then climb to the top of the monkey bars. They just go out there and fool around and play and do whatever they feel like doing.

By saying this, I don't mean to suggest that having sexual intercourse is like going out to the playground to fool around (although there is a certain playfulness that can happen when two people are having sex). The point is that there just aren't any specific rules or instructions, or one "right way," to have sexual intercourse.

Some people like to hug and kiss a lot first. Touching, kissing, and hugging usually give people warm, excited, sexual feelings. The couple may then touch, rub, or caress each other's genitals or breasts before intercourse, which is called *foreplay*. They may also engage in oral-genital sex. *Oral-genital sex*, which is also called oral sex, or in slang terms "69-ing" or "a blow job," involves people using their mouths to stimulate each other's genital organs.

When questions about oral-genital sex come up in the class question box and I explain what it is, many kids go, "Oh, yuck, why would anyone want to do that? I explain that many couples find this a very pleasurable way of enjoying each other's bodies and a special way of being close. It's also a way of being sexual with someone that doesn't involve the possibility of the woman's getting pregnant. Many kids find the idea of oral-genital sex kind of revolting because they think of this area of the body as being "dirty" or full of germs. Actually, though, this area of our bodies isn't any dirtier or more germ-laden than other parts of our bodies. In fact, most people's mouths have more germs than their genitals.

Another thing that bothers some young people when they hear about something like oral-genital sex is that they think that it's something you *have* to do when you have sex. This isn't true. Some couples enjoy oral-genital sex and often include it in their lovemaking. Others have religious or moral objections to it, or don't feel comfortable with it, so they don't do it. It's normal if you do and normal if you don't. Like everything else about sex, you're the one who decides what you do or don't want to do, and you never have to do anything that doesn't seem right for you.

Is sex painful for women?

No, sex isn't painful for women, or for men either. In fact, sex usually feels quite wonderful, provided of course that the two partners feel good about what they are doing, care about each other, and are considerate of each other's feelings.

As we've explained, the penis gets thicker and wider when it's erect, but the vagina is a very stretchy and elastic organ and easily expands to accommodate an erect penis. When a male is sexually aroused ("turned on"), his penis produces a small amount of lubricating fluid. When a female is sexually aroused, her vagina also produces lubricating fluid. These fluids help the penis slide into the vagina comfortably. In addition, the upper portion of the vagina also "balloons out" or expands somewhat when a female becomes sexually aroused, so there's usually no discomfort when the penis goes into the vagina.

If, however, a couple tries to have sex before the female is fully aroused and her vagina has begun to lubricate and expand, having sex could be uncomfortable. Since males sometimes become aroused more quickly than females, it's important for the couple to make sure that the female has enough foreplay so she is ready and well-lubricated before the penis enters the vagina.

Although sex isn't usually painful, when a female

has sex for the first time (or for the first several times), she sometimes experiences some discomfort or pain. This may happen for any of a number of reasons. For one thing, she may be nervous, which makes her tighten her vaginal muscles and decreases the lubrication in her vagina. Or both partners may be rushing things, trying to put the penis into the vagina before she's lubricated enough. If the female is a virgin (a person who's never had sex before), her vaginal opening or the opening in her hymen may be rather small and tight. If the couple doesn't go slowly and gently, the hymen or vaginal opening can be painfully stretched or torn. This is why it is important for a couple to begin their sex lives in a relaxed and gentle manner.

How does it feel to have sex?

I get asked this question a lot and to tell you the truth, it's hard to answer. Sex feels different to different people. But, most people agree that it feels wonderful.

Of course, how it feels depends a lot on the situation. If you're having sex with someone you love and the two of you both feel comfortable about what you're doing, then sex can bring pleasure, fun, passion, and joy. There's a rush of good feeling when you share a good sexual experience with someone you truly care about. Sex can be a very special way of being close to someone and of discovering more about each other.

But sex can also bring sadness and emotional pain. If you don't truly care about each other or you don't feel it's right for you to be having sex, intercourse may not be a pleasant feeling at all. If you're wondering about how you'd know if it was right for you, you might read the section entitled "Making Decisions About How to Handle Your Romantic and Sexual Feelings" in the last chapter.

PREGNANCY AND CHILDBIRTH

Questions about pregnancy and childbirth often come up in class. Here are some of the questions that have been asked.

Are there only certain times of the month when a girl can get pregnant, and if so, when?

Yes, the ovum can be fertilized only during the thirty-six or so hours (some experts say forty-eight hours) right after it has left the ovary, because only then is it at the exact ripeness to allow for fertilization. After that, the egg is "overripe" and cannot be fertilized. Within a few days, it will break down and disintegrate completely.

Because there's only, at most, forty-eight hours during which an ovum can be fertilized in each menstrual cycle, it would seem to be a pretty easy thing to avoid getting pregnant: just don't have sex during those forty-eight hours. Unfortunately, it's not that simple. First of all, sperm can stay alive in the female's body for up to three (some experts say five) days. So, let's say a woman ovulated on the 10th day of the month. If she'd had sex on the 7th and the man had ejaculated, the sperm could still be in her body, alive and well, waiting for the ovum when it popped off the ovary on the 10th.

Also, there's no way to predict ahead of time exactly when a female is going to ovulate. A female usually ovulates twelve to sixteen days before the first day of bleeding of her next menstrual period. So we can count backwards and get an idea of when she ovulated in the previous cycle. But we *can't* tell when she'll ovulate in the next cycle because, as we've explained, menstrual cycles aren't always regular. One month, the cycle may last twenty-eight days, the next month thirty-two, and the next twenty-one. Even females who have fairly regular periods, say every twenty-seven or twenty-eight days, will occasionally have cycles that are longer or shorter than usual. So, even though there is only a short time during each month when a female can get pregnant, it's impossible to tell exactly when that time will come.

I heard that if you only have sex during your period, you won't get pregnant. Is this true?

No, females can and do become pregnant from having sex while they're having their menstrual period. A female whose period lasts for longer than seven days is more likely to get pregnant from having sex during her period. But, even a female whose period lasts seven days or less could get pregnant from having sex during this time.

Here's an example of how this might work. Say Mary starts her period on June 3rd. She bleeds for seven days, until June 9th. She has sex on June 8th, while she's still bleeding. Her next period starts on June 24th. Altogether, twenty-one days have elapsed between the first day of bleeding of her period on June 3rd and the first day of bleeding of her next period on June 24th. By counting back twelve to sixteen days from June 24th, we can figure that she probably ovulated between June 8th and June 12th. Mary was still bleeding on the 8th; she may have ovulated on the 8th; she had sex on the 8th. So, there is a chance she could get pregnant, even though she was having her period.

Even if Mary didn't ovulate until the 9th or 10th, she still might get pregnant because sperm can stay alive for at least three days. And if the experts who say that sperm can stay alive for five days are right, she might have gotten pregnant from having sex on the 8th, even if she didn't ovulate until the 12th.

Let's look at another example. Susan begins her period on August lst. She bleeds for seven days, until August 7th. She has sex on August 7th, while she's still bleeding. Her next period starts on August 28th, which means she had a twenty-seven-day cycle. So she may have ovulated as early as August 12th. Even though she stopped bleeding on the 7th, there might still be some live sperm in her body from the time she had sex on the 7th. Therefore, if Susan ovulated on August 12th, she could have become pregnant from having had sex on the 7th while she was still menstruating.

So it is possible for a female to get pregnant from having sex during her menstrual period.

How old does a girl have to be before she can get pregnant? Could a girl ever get pregnant before she'd had her first period?
Once a girl reaches puberty and begins to menstruate and ovulate, she is physically capable of becoming pregnant. As we explained in Chapter 6 (see pages 130–132), it would be *highly* unlikely, in fact next to impossible, for a girl to get pregnant before she'd had her first period.

Can a girl get pregnant the first time she has sex?
Yes, girls can and do get pregnant, even if they've only had sex one time.

Does a girl have to have sexual intercourse to get pregnant?
Generally speaking, the answer is yes. But even if the male didn't actually put his penis in her vagina, it would be possible for her to become pregnant if the sperm

were ejaculated *near* the opening of the vagina. The sperm could swim into the vagina, up into the uterus, and into the fallopian tube, where it could fertilize the ovum. Also, even if a male were to pull his penis out of the vagina and ejaculate in such a way that none of the sperm got into the vagina or near the vaginal opening, pregnancy might still occur. As a male gets sexually aroused and his penis gets erect, a few drops of seminal fluid often appear at the tip of his penis. This fluid may contain sperm, and these sperm could cause pregnancy.

We should mention that, no matter what you've heard, a female *can't* get pregnant from kissing, masturbating herself, swimming in a pool, sitting on someone's lap, or sitting on a toilet seat. In fact, with the exception of special medical procedures that doctors use to help women who are having problems getting pregnant, there are no ways in which a female can become pregnant other than the ones we've mentioned here.

Are there some people who aren't able to have babies?
Yes. Some men and women are *infertile* or *sterile*, which means they aren't able to reproduce. A number of things can cause infertility. In females, infertility is often the result of scar tissue from past infections of the reproductive organs (see the section on pelvic inflammatory disease on page 178). The scar tissue may prevent ovulation, block the fallopian tubes so the ovum can't travel

infertile (in-FER-tull)
sterile (STEH-rull)
infertility (in-fer-TILL-uh-tee)
sterility (stuh-RILL-uh-tee)

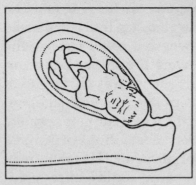

The cervix is fully dilated

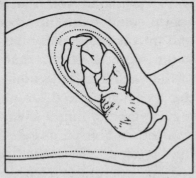

The baby's head moves into the vagina

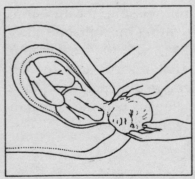

The baby's head comes out of the vagina

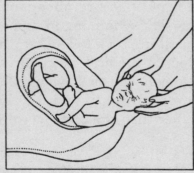

The baby's shoulders follow

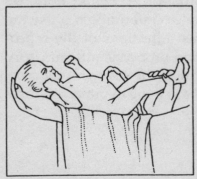

After the birth, the umbilical cord is clamped

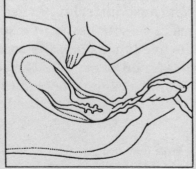

Afterward, the placenta is also pushed out of the uterus

Illustration 31. The Birth Process

to the uterus, or otherwise prevent the reproductive organs from working properly. Hormone imbalances and certain diseases of the ovary can also prevent ovulation. Medical problems affecting the uterus and tubes can cause infertility, too.

In males, infertility is usually due to one of the following: too few sperm being produced, sperm that can't swim properly or are otherwise abnormal, or a blockage in the testicles or vas deferens which prevents the sperm from getting to the penis. These problems may be the result of a twisted vein in the testicle, hormonal imbalances, exposure to X-rays, drugs or other harmful substances, past infections, or other medical problems.

In many cases, infertility can be treated by medicines or surgery, but this isn't always possible.

How old is a woman before she's too old to have a baby?

Women stop having babies when they've gone through *menopause*. Menopause is the time in a woman's life when her ovaries stop producing a ripe ovum each month and she stops having her menstrual periods. It usually happens between the ages of forty-five and fifty-five, although it can happen earlier or later for some women.

As far as we know, the oldest woman who ever had a baby was a fifty-six-year-old grandmother from Glendale, California. Although her periods were coming only once in a while, the woman had not yet gone through menopause. She had sexual intercourse, and much to her surprise, she got pregnant. She gave birth to a normal, healthy baby.

Why are some babies girls and some boys?

The sex of the baby depends on the father's sperm. Some sperm have what scientists call an "x" chromosome, which means they are capable of uniting with an ovum and making a female baby. Other sperm have a *"y"* chromosome, which means that they are capable of uniting with an ovum and making a male baby. If a *y*-factor sperm fertilizes the ovum, the baby will be a boy; if an *x*-factor sperm fertilizes the ovum, the baby will be a girl.

How long does pregnancy take?
Females are usually pregnant for about nine months; however, sometimes pregnancy can last a little longer or a little less than this. If the baby is born at only eight months or earlier, we say the baby is "premature." Many premature babies are perfectly normal and healthy; others need special medical care. If a baby is born very prematurely, before six months or so, its chances of surviving are much lower. If a pregnancy lasts much more than nine months, the doctor may give the woman medication to make the baby come because it isn't healthy for the baby to stay in the uterus too long.

What happens when a baby is born?
When a baby is ready to be born, the mother goes into what we call *labor*. During labor, the muscles of the mother's uterus begin to contract rhythmically and the mother feels a cramping sensation. At first, the contractions aren't very strong and only come once in awhile. As labor continues, the contractions become stronger and stronger and come more often. At some point during labor or childbirth, the *amniotic sac*, the bag of fluids inside which the baby grows, breaks open, and the woman feels a gushing or leaking of fluid from her vagina. If the amniotic sac doesn't break on its own, the doctor will break it.

chromosome (CROW-moe-soam)
amniotic (AM-knee-OT-ik)

During labor, the opening of the cervix, the lower portion of the uterus that protrudes into the vagina, also begins to *dilate* (open up). When the cervix is fully dilated and the contractions are strong and regular, the force of the contractions begins to push the baby out of the uterus, through the cervix, through the vagina, and out the vaginal opening (see Illustration 31). Most babies are born head first, but some babies come out feet first or with some other part of the baby coming first. The average length of labor time for woman's first baby is about twelve to fourteen hours, and about seven hours for subsequent pregnancies.

For some women, labor and childbirth is very painful; for others there is little or no pain. But for most women, there is some discomfort, since the contractions have to be very strong in order to push the baby out. Some women practice certain exercises before pregnancy and use breathing techniques during labor which help control the pain. If the pain is too intense, the woman may choose to have an anesthetic, often one which numbs her from the waist down so she doesn't feel the pain.

Once labor has progressed to the point where the cervix is fully dilated (opened to about 4 inches), the "pushing stage" of labor begins. During this stage, the mother, if she hasn't been anesthetized, can bear down or push along with the contractions and help bring the baby out. Even if she can't help by pushing, the contractions alone are usually enough to push the baby out into the world. If not, the doctor can reach inside and help move the baby out.

This pushing stage usually lasts for one-half hour to three hours with a first pregnancy, and for about a half-

dilate (DIE-late)
anesthetic (an-ess-THET-ik)
anesthetized (an-ESS-theh-TIZED)

hour with subsequent pregnancies, but it may be shorter or longer than this.

During the pushing stage, the baby begins to move out of the uterus and through the cervix into the vagina. Once the entire top of the baby's head is visible at the vaginal opening, things happen very quickly. It usually only takes a few more contractions to push the baby out entirely.

When a baby is born it has a cord, known as the *umbilical cord*, attached to its belly button. The other end of this cord is attached to the *placenta*. The placenta is a special organ that develops inside the uterus during pregnancy to bring blood and nourishment from the mother to the baby. The placenta usually comes out within a half-hour after the baby. The doctor then cuts the cord and disposes of it and the placenta. The cord is cut within a couple of inches of the baby's belly button and is clamped or tied closed. By the time the baby is a few weeks old, the cord will have dried up and fallen off by itself.

After birth, the doctor or nurse checks the baby to make sure it's breathing property, and may clean it up a bit before giving it to its mother to hold. The boys and girls in my class get a big kick out of hearing about their own births. You might ask your mother to tell you about her labor with you.

What is a Cesarean section?
If for one reason or another, a baby can't be born through the vaginal canal, the doctor does an operation called

umbilical (um-BILL-i-KUL)
placenta (pla-SEN-ta)
Cesarean (si-ZARE-ee-en)

a *Cesarean* section, or C-section. The woman is anesthetized, so she can't feel anything from her waist down. The doctor makes an incision in her abdomen and uterus and removes the baby from her body by lifting it out through the incision. Afterwards, the incision is sewn shut. Babies born by C-section are usually perfectly healthy.

There are a number of reasons why a baby might have to be born by C-section. For example, labor may be taking so long that the baby is getting worn out and it's heartbeat is slowing down. Or the baby might be in a position that would make a vaginal delivery difficult or impossible. The woman's cervix might not be dilating properly or her contractions might be too weak to push the baby out. For these or other reasons, the doctor might need to do a C-section.

What is an embryo? What's a fetus?

After an ovum has been fertilized and has planted itself in the uterus, it begins the nine-month process of developing into a baby. For the first three months, it is referred to as an *embryo*. After three months, it is called a *fetus*.

What is a miscarriage? What is a stillbirth?

When an embryo or fetus dies, it is expelled from the mother's uterus and this is called *miscarriage*. Most miscarriages happen during the first three months of pregnancy, but they can happen later in pregnancy, too.

embryo (EM-bree-oh)
fetus (FEE-tus)
miscarriage (MISS-care-ij)

Doctors aren't always sure why a miscarriage has happened, but usually the embryo or fetus has a defect or problem in its development that makes it impossible for it to survive. Having a miscarriage doesn't usually affect a woman's chances of having a normal baby in the future.

Stillbirth means that the baby is born dead. In some cases, the baby has died during the birth process; in other cases, the baby has died in the uterus shortly before birth. Sometimes the doctor can figure out why it happened; at other times it's a complete mystery. Fortunately, stillbirths and miscarriages after the third month of pregnancy are very rare. The vast majority of women have normal pregnancies and give birth to healthy babies.

What are birth defects and why do they happen?
Sometimes babies are born with medical problems such as blindness, brain damage, heart or lung problems, deformed limbs, or other birth defects. Birth defects may be caused by defects in the ovum or sperm, inherited problems from the mother or father, the mother being exposed to harmful drugs or X-rays during pregnancy, a disease the mother has contracted during pregnancy, premature birth, or problems with the baby not getting enough oxygen right after birth. There are also other, less common causes, and sometimes the cause of a birth defect is not known. Fortunately, birth defects are very rare, and most babies are born completely healthy.

How do twins happen? How come twins don't always look alike? If a woman has twins, do they both come out at the same time?
Twins can happen in one of two ways: either there are two fertilized ova, or there is one fertilized ovum that splits in two (see Illustration 32).

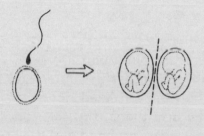

Sometimes a woman will produce two ripe ova the same month. If each of these ova is fertilized by sperm, the woman will have fraternal twins.

At other times, a sperm may fertilize a single ripe ovum. Then, after fertilization, the ovum splits into two, and the woman will have identical twins.

Illustration 32. Twins

Usually a woman's ovaries produce only one ripe ovum a month. Occasionally, though, a woman will produce two ripe ova at the same time. If both of these ova are fertilized and plant themselves in the lining of the uterus, the woman will have twins. Twins that grow from two separate ova, fertilized by two separate sperm, are called *fraternal* twins. With fraternal twins, one may be a boy and one a girl, or they may both be the same sex. They won't necessarily look alike.

fraternal (frah-TUR-nul)

The other type of twins is called *identical* twins. Identical twins happen when a fertilized ovum splits in two shortly after fertilization. No one knows why this happens. Twins that come from the same ovum and sperm look alike and are always the same sex.

When twins are born, one baby comes out first and the other comes out within a few minutes. In some cases, it takes more than a few minutes for the second twin to be born. There have even been cases where it took a whole day. But, usually, twins are born within a few minutes of each other.

What are Siamese twins?

Siamese twins are identical twins who are born with their bodies attached to each other in some way. Siamese twins happen when the fertilized ovum is splitting in two, making identical twins. But for some unknown reason, the split is not completed and the babies develop so that some parts of their bodies are joined together.

Identical twins are pretty rare. Siamese twins are even rarer. When Siamese twins do happen, they may be joined in a number of ways—at the feet, the shoulders, or the arms. When they are attached in such places, they are generally fairly easy to separate. A doctor can operate (usually shortly after the babies are born) and cut the babies apart. But sometimes it's not so easy. The babies may be joined at the head or chest or in such a way that cutting them apart would kill one or both of them. The parents may decide to have the operation done even though one baby will die. If the parents decide not to have the operation, or if it's not possible to operate without killing both babies, the twins spend their lives attached to each other.

What about triplets? What are the most babies a woman ever had at one time?

Triplets (three babies), quadruplets (four), quintuplets (five), sextuplets (six), septuplets (seven), and octuplets (eight) happen much less frequently than twins.

Whenever more than three babies are born at one time, the chances of all the babies surviving is lower. Because there are so many of them, they're smaller than normal babies, and they're usually born prematurely, that is, before they've had a chance to develop fully. As far as we know, the largest number of babies born at one time is twelve, but not all of them survived; the largest number that ever lived was eight, or possibly nine.

Nowadays, doctors have drugs, called *fertility drugs*, that they give to women who haven't been able to get pregnant because they don't ovulate. These drugs stimulate the ovaries and cause the woman to ovulate. The problem is that they can stimulate the ovaries so much that the woman produces not one but several ripe ova at the same time.

BIRTH CONTROL

If two people want to have intercourse, but they don't want to become pregnant, they must use birth control. Birth control is also called *contraception* or *family planning*, and there are several different types or methods.

A lot of teens are getting pregnant these days—about 3,000 a day, or over a million each year. Experts estimate that four out of every ten of today's 14-year-old girls will have been pregnant at least once by the end of their teen years. So I spend a lot of time talking about birth control in my classes for older kids.

contraception (KON-treh-SEP-shen)

Even in my youngest classes, where most of the kids haven't yet started to go through puberty, I still spend at least some time talking about birth control. I think that starting to learn about contraception long before you might actually have a need for it is a good idea. That way, birth control becomes less mysterious, something you're used to hearing about as you grow older. When you do eventually become sexually active, you won't have to learn about birth control for the first time.

This section will help you start learning some of the basic facts about contraception. Of course, as you grow older, you'll need more information than is given here. Some of the books listed on pages 242–245 will help you learn more about contraception. If you are already sexually active or are thinking about having sex in the near future, you probably need more information than you'll find in this or any other book. You might want to visit your local Planned Parenthood clinic. They have special birth control classes for teens, and their nurses and doctors are experienced in helping young people choose a method. (Look under "Planned Parenthood" in the white pages, under "Family Planning" in the yellow pages, or call the information operator.)

Of course, any family planning clinic or private doctor can help you learn about or obtain a method of birth control. And, anyone, regardless of their age, can get a prescription for or purchase any method of birth control. You don't need parental permission, and doctors are not required to notify your parents. So please don't hesitate to get the protection you need.

Methods of Birth Control

Most contraceptive methods currently in use work in one or more of the following ways: 1) by preventing ovulation, 2) by preventing fertilization, or 3) by altering the lining of the uterus so a fertilized ovum is prevented from growing there.

The most common methods are listed below. Most methods are "female" methods because they are used by and affect the female, but the condom and male sterilization are "male" methods. Some methods require a doctor's prescription, but many (the sponge, spermicides, and condoms) can be purchased at drug stores, and even some grocery stores without a prescription.

Most of these methods are "temporary," meaning that once you stop using them, pregnancy is again possible. However, the last method listed—sterilization—is considered permanent because it is usually impossible for a person who's been sterilized to ever become pregnant again.

1. *Birth Control Pills:* A monthly series of hormone pills which protect against pregnancy as long as they are taken according to schedule. However, forgetting to take even one pill may result in pregnancy.
2. *The Intrauterine Device (IUD):* A soft plastic device which is inserted into the uterus by a doctor and which may be left in place up to several years, depending on the type of used. The IUD should only be removed by a doctor—never by the woman herself. Because of safety hazards, the IUD is no longer manufactured in the US.
3. *The Diaphragm:* A soft rubber dome that is filled with a spermicide (sperm-killing chemical) and inserted into the vagina before sexual intercourse. If at least eight hours have passed since intercourse, the device can then be removed, cleaned, and stored for future use.
4. *The Cervical Cap:* Also used with spermicides, the cap is inserted, removed, and stored just like the diaphragm. The main difference is that the cap is smaller, shaped differently, covers only the cervix, and is held in place by suction.

intrauterine (In-trah-YOU-ter-in)
diaphragm (DIE-eh-FRAM)

5. *The Contraceptive Sponge:* Similar in size and shape to a powder puff, the sponge is moistened with water to release its spermicide and inserted into the top of the vagina before sex. It is used once and then thrown away.

6. *Spermicides:* May come in the form of creams or jellies which are used alone or with a cap or diaphragm: tablets, which dissolve when placed in the vagina; or aerosol foams, which are inserted into the vagina before sex by means of a special applicator.

7. *Condoms* ("rubbers"): A tube of thin rubber that fits over the erect penis like a glove over a finger. Held in place by a band of rubber at its lower edge, the condom traps semen inside. It is only used once and then thrown away. Most condoms come rolled up, in foil packets. If there isn't a "reservoir tip," one-half inch of space must be left at the top of the condom to allow room for the semen to collect. Otherwise, the semen could be forced down the sides of the penis and out the lower edge of the condom.

8. *The Rhythm Method:* Involves keeping track of the female's menstrual periods on a calendar and not having sex around the time of ovulation, when she is most likely to become pregnant. Because it is so difficult to guess when ovulation will occur (see pages 150–151), this is not a very effective method of birth control.

9. *Natural Family Planning (NFP):* An improvement on the rhythm method. Instead of just counting on a calendar, people who use NFP also keep charts of the female's daily body temperature and the type of mucous secreted by her cervix, which is a more accurate way of determining ovulation. Thus, NFP is much more effective than the rhythm method. Intercourse must be avoided on certain days with both rhythm and NFP.

10. *The Morning After Pill (MAP):* An emergency method which is only used when a female has had sex without the protection of birth control. The pills must be taken within 72 hours after sex in order to work. Because the dose of hormones is so high, this cannot be used as a regular method of birth control.

condom (KON-dem)
spermicide (SPURM-eh-SIDE)

11. *Injectable Contraceptive:* A high dose of hormone injected into a female's body. The hormone is slowly released into the body. A single shot can prevent pregnancy for up to three months. (Not used in the United States, see page 170.)

12. *Abortion:* Used when people become pregnant but don't want to keep the baby or give it up for adoption. Abortions are usually done before the fourteenth week of pregnancy. An anesthetic is given and one end of a small suction tube is inserted through the vagina, and into the uterus. The other end of the tube is attached to a vacuum machine. The bloody menstrual lining and the developing pregnancy are then gently sucked out through the tube. Although abortions may be done up to the twenty-fourth week, these later abortions are more complicated and may have to be done in a hospital or clinic rather than at a doctor's office.

13. *Male or Female Sterilization:* An operation which in men is called *vasectomy* and in women *tubal ligation* or "tying the tubes." The vas deferens (the tube through which sperm travel from the testicles to the penis) or the fallopian tubes are cut, tied, sealed, or otherwise blocked off so pregnancy can't occur. Afterwards, the body keeps producing sperm and ova, but they are reabsorbed by the body.

Effectiveness

Although no birth control method is 100% effective, most of those listed here are highly effective, provided they are used correctly, *exactly according to instructions*. However, the rhythm method, the sponge, and spermicidal tablets, jellies, or creams used on their own (without a cap or a diaphragm) are the least effective. People who absolutely don't want to become pregnant should not use these methods.

You sometimes hear that methods like the pill and the IUD are more effective than condoms. Actually,

sterilization (STARE-eh-leh-ZAY-shen)
abortion (uh-BORE-shen)
vasectomy (vas-EK-teh-me)
ligation (leh-GAY-shen)

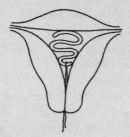

The IUD inside the uterus

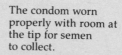

The condom worn properly with room at the tip for semen to collect.

The condom

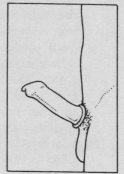

MON	TUES	WED	THUR	FRI	SAT	SUN
		1	2	3	4	5
6	7	8	~~9~~	~~10~~	~~11~~	~~12~~
~~13~~	~~14~~	15	16	17	18	19
20	21	22	23	24	25	26
27	28	29	30			

The rhythm method and Natural Family Planning (NFP) involve keeping track of the female's menstrual periods to determine when she will be ovulating.

Illustration 33. Types of Birth Control

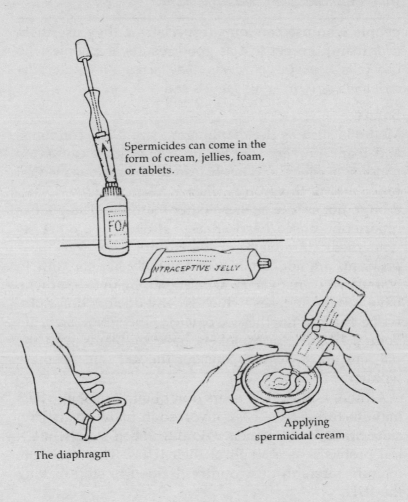

Spermicides can come in the form of cream, jellies, foam, or tablets.

Applying spermicidal cream

The diaphragm

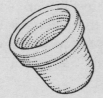

The cervical cap

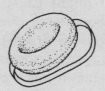

The contraceptive sponge

people who use condoms (especially if they use them *with* foam) can get just as good results as people who use pills, *provided, of course, that they are used properly, each and every time a person has sex.*

Safety

Methods such as the diaphragm, cap, NFP, condoms, and foam are very safe because they don't cause any major side effects and rarely lead to any serious medical problems. Birth control pills are also considered safe, though not as safe as these other methods. The pill has reportedly caused heart attacks, strokes, and other serious medical problems in some users. However, these problems are not common and usually happen only in women who are over 35, who smoke cigarettes, or who have certain diseases (which is why doctors don't prescribe the pill for these women). Only *very* rarely do young, healthy, nonsmokers have problems with the pill, and most doctors consider the pill safe for these women.

Although most IUD users don't have problems, IUD manufacturers have been involved in many costly lawsuits brought by women who developed serious medical problems as a result of their IUDs. Therefore, the manufacturers in this country decided to stop making the IUD.

Some doctors are concerned that the injectable contraceptive might cause cancer or infertility in some women. Because of questions about the safety of this method, our government has not approved the injectable contraceptive for use in the United States, though it is available in many other countries.

Choosing a Method

Choosing a type of birth control involves weighing the relative effectiveness, convenience, and safety of each method. A couple's choice will also depend on many other factors including: the female's health, her age, the state of the couple's relationship, and whether they just want to "space" pregnancies or absolutely don't want to become pregnant. Most people use several different methods over the course of their lives.

Many young people begin by using a condom. The condom is easy to obtain and can protect against some sexually transmitted diseases (see pages 184–185). Later, they may switch to one of the methods that require a doctor's prescription. Some couples prefer methods such as the IUD or pill because they don't like to interrupt their lovemaking by having to put on a condom, diaphragm, or cap or to use spermicides. However, women who don't have intercourse very often may choose one of these methods rather than the pill, which must be taken regularly, or an IUD, which is in place constantly. Women who are concerned about the side effects of the pill or the IUD may choose one of the safer methods. Men or women who have completed their families may choose sterilization.

The boys and girls in my class often ask lots of questions about birth control—more than we have space for here. However, there is one method in particular that they have questions about—abortion. As you may know, abortion is a very controversial topic, so in the rest of this section we're going to answer some of the questions that my students ask about abortion.

What's wrong with not using birth control and just having an abortion if you get pregnant?
Different people would answer this question somewhat differently. Some people feel that abortion is morally wrong, that it is the same as murder, and that it should be outlawed. They feel that a pregnant woman should have her baby and either keep the child or put it up

for adoption. Since these people feel that abortion is morally wrong, they would, of course, feel that using abortion as a regular method of contraception (or, indeed, even once) is not okay.

Other people feel that abortion is a private matter between a woman and her doctor, and that a woman should have the right to decide what goes on inside her body, including whether or not she wants to have a baby. But even people who feel abortion is morally acceptable often feel that it's just not right or ethical for a person to rely on abortion as a regular method of birth control. They feel that abortion should only be used as a "back-up" measure when the regular method has failed to prevent pregnancy and the woman doesn't want to continue the pregnancy.

Aside from the moral and ethical reasons, there are also good medical reasons why people shouldn't have abortions whenever they become pregnant. If a woman didn't use contraception, she'd probably find herself getting pregnant at least once a year, if not more often. Having abortions this often could lead to serious medical problems.

How would a girl know whether or not she was pregnant?
Most females discover that they are pregnant because they fail to have their menstrual period at the expected time. Sore breasts and nausea are also early signs of pregnancy. There are many reasons other than pregnancy that could cause these symptoms, but pregnancy is the most common cause of missed periods in sexually active females. Anyone who thinks she might be pregnant should have a pregnancy test.

Standard pregnancy tests are done on a urine sample collected in the early morning. In order for some tests to be accurate, at least fourteen days must have elapsed since the time of the expected menstrual period—that is, the female must be at least fourteen days "late" in getting her period. There are also tests that can detect pregnancy earlier, that is, before the female is fourteen days late in getting her period. Standard pregnancy tests are available from private doctors or family planning clinics such as Planned Parenthood.

In addition, do-it-yourself pregnancy test kits are available at drug stores. If a person follows the directions exactly, these tests are quite reliable. However, it is possible to get a false test result. If the home pregnancy test indicates a female isn't pregnant, but she still doesn't get her period, or she has other signs of pregnancy, or if she feels unsure about the test results, she should have a test done at a doctor's office or clinic.

What if the test shows that you are pregnant?

If pregnancy occurs, there are three choices: 1) continuing the pregnancy and keeping the baby, 2) continuing the pregnancy but giving the child up for adoption, and 3) abortion. If you are not certain which is the best choice for you, the doctor at the place where you got your pregnancy test can refer you to a counselor who will help you decide. Regardless of what decision you make, you have the right to sympathetic counseling and to complete information about each of the choices available. Even if you feel certain about your decision, you may find it helpful to discuss your decision with a member of your family or a counselor.

Does a girl need her parent's permission to get an abortion? How much does it cost? Where can you get an abortion?

A girl doesn't need her parent's permission in order to have an abortion, regardless of her age. Abortions can be done in doctor's offices, hospitals, or clinics. They usually cost anywhere from $150 and $1000, depending on the type of abortion and when it is done. If a girl can't afford to pay for an abortion, Planned Parenthood clinics can provide abortion services or referrals for free or low-cost abortions. State or county welfare offices can also provide this information (ask the information operator for the state or county Welfare Department or the Department of Human and Social Services).

After we've talked about intercourse, pregnancy and childbirth, and birth control in class, we usually move on to the topic of sexually transmitted diseases, and then to other sexual health issues. There isn't any special reason why we move from one topic to the next in this order, but since that's usually how it happens, in the next chapter we'll discuss these topics in pretty much the same order that we do in class.

CHAPTER 8

Sexually Transmitted Diseases, AIDS, and Other Sexual Health Issues

One day not long ago, the kids in my fifth-grade class and I were going through the class question box. I pulled out a folded scrap of paper which had these two questions written on it:

What is BD?
What is Ben Aerial's disease and what does it have to do with sex?

At first, I didn't have a clue as to what these questions were about. I just stood there, staring at the paper and mumbling to myself: "BD? . . . Ben Aerial? . . . like the aerial antenna on a television set? . . . *Ben Aerial's disease??* . . . What in the world???"

Then all of a sudden I realized what had happened: The student who wrote these questions had apparently overheard some people talking and thought they were saying *BD* when it was really *VD* they were talking about. This kid wanted to find out about *venereal disease* (not Ben Aerial's disease!), which is a group of diseases people can get from having sex.

In the first section of this chapter, we'll be talking about these diseases. However, because VD is a sort of old-fashioned term, we'll be using the more modern term, "sexually transmitted diseases," or STDs.

You may notice that we haven't included AIDS, an STD that's been in the news a lot lately, in the section on STDs. That's because AIDS is different from the other STDs in several important ways; therefore, we decided to discuss AIDS in a separate section of its own.

The AIDS section follows the STD section. In addition, there are two other sections in this chapter that deal with health problems related to the sex organs or sexual activity. We hope this chapter helps answer any questions you may have about these sexual health issues.

SEXUALLY TRANSMITTED DISEASES (STDs)

Each year more than a million teenagers in the United States develop an STD. Since these diseases are usually transmitted sexually, kids who haven't started having sex yet don't really need to worry about STDs. Still, we think it never hurts to start learning about them while you're still young. Besides, kids are often curious about this topic, so even in my classes for younger kids, we spend some time talking about STDs.

In this section we'll be explaining the basic facts about STDs. If, however, you'd like more information than is given here, you'll find some helpful books in the Further Reading list in the back of this book. You can also call the National VD Hotline (see page 184) for information about STDs.

Symptoms

There are more than twenty different types of STDs. Although each type has its own particular symptoms, generally speaking, STDs cause the following kinds of symptoms:

- An unusual discharge from the penis or vagina.
- Itching, burning, redness, rashes, lumps, bumps, or sores in, on, or around the sex organs.
- Pain or tenderness in the sex organs, the genital area, or the lower abdomen.
- Burning or pain when urinating, or a frequent need to urinate.

These symptoms can also be caused by diseases that aren't sexually transmitted, but any sexually active person who develops these symptoms needs to see a doctor in order to be tested for STDs, and if necessary, treated.

It is possible to have an STD but not have any symptoms or have only mild, temporary symptoms that clear up on their own, without treatment. Nonetheless, the germs may still be in the body, which means the person is still capable of passing the disease to other people.

Types of STDs

Syphilis is an STD that was a dreaded disease back before antibiotics had been discovered. The germs would spread from the sex organs to the brain, heart, lungs, and other organs, causing insanity and/or death. Nowadays, though, syphilis can be treated with antibiotics before it has a chance to spread.

Gonorrhea and *chlamydia* are two very common STDs which are serious problems for females because, unlike males, females often don't have any symptoms and,

syphilis (SIF-eh-lis)
gonorrhea (GONE-ah-REE-uh)
chlamydia (KLUH-mid-ee-uh)

therefore, don't seek treatment. Thus, the germs may remain in the vagina. Then, weeks, months, or even years later, the germs may move upwards, spreading the infection to the uterus, fallopian tubes, and ovaries. Infection of these organs, known as *pelvic inflammatory disease* (PID), can be a very serious type of STD. It often requires a hospital stay, and in some cases, it may be necessary to operate and remove the infected organs. Even if there are no symptoms or only mild ones, PID can seriously damage these organs, causing infertility or life-long recurrences of the infection, as well as other major health problems.

Genital warts and *genital herpes*, which are also very common, are both caused by viruses. Here again, these STDs can be especially serious for females because these viruses sometimes lead to cancer of the cervix. Herpes can also cause miscarriages, premature births, and other problems during childbirth and pregnancy. In fact, herpes, whose chief symptom is painful, blister-like sores, can be serious for both males and females because, unlike other STDs, herpes is incurable. Once you get it, the virus remains in your body for the rest of your life. But this doesn't mean you'll always have the sores. After a few weeks, the viruses retreat deep into the body and the sores disappear and the person is no longer capable of infecting others. However, the viruses usually surface from time to time, causing new outbreaks of the sores and other symptoms. During these outbreaks, and for a time before and after, the person is again capable of passing the virus on to his or her sex partner.

Not all STDs are this serious. For instance, *tricho-*

herpes (HER-peez)
trichomoniasis (TRICK-o-moan-EYE-uh-sis)

moniasis (trich or TV), *candidiasis* (yeast infections), and *Gardnerella* (Hemophilus) can cause bothersome symptoms, but they rarely, if ever, lead to major medical problems. In fact, although males may pass these infections to their female sex partners, they themselves don't usually develop any symptoms. The same is true of *nonspecific vaginitis*, an STDs that affects females. "Vaginitis" means inflammation of the vagina and "nonspecific" means the doctor can't find any specific germ that's causing the infection.

Nonspecific urethritis (NSU) is another infection that is often (though not always) transmitted sexually. "Urethritis" means inflammation of the urethra and "nonspecific" means the doctor can't pinpoint a specific germ that is causing the urinary symptoms. NSU is more common in males than in females. Although NSU can lead to *cystitis* (infections of the bladder) and other more serious kidney or urinary tract infections, it is usually treated before these problems occur. Thus, NSU isn't considered as serious as some of the other STDs.

Pubic lice, or "crabs," is perhaps the least serious of all the STDs, though it's certainly no fun having them. The lice are tiny, crab-like, bloodsucking insects that can be found in the pubic hair, head hair, and sometimes the eyelashes. Their bite causes intense itching that is often worse at night. Getting rid of lice involves repeated shampoos with a special lotion, and dry cleaning or boiling all bed linen, undergarments, and any other infected clothing (or stuffing them in a plastic bag for two weeks) to make sure all the lice are dead.

candidiasis (CAN-di-DIE-uh-sis)
Gardnerella (GARD-ner-ELL-uh)
Hemophilus (he-MOF-eh-lus)
vaginitis (VAJ-en-NI-tis)
urethritis (YOUR-rith-RYE-tis)
cystitis (sis-TIE-tis)

How STDs Are Spread

Most STDs are caused by germs that can only survive in the moist, mucous membranes of the human body, that is, in places like the penis, vulva, vagina, rectum, mouth, or throat. Most of the germs die almost immediately when exposed to air. However, certain STD germs, such as trichs, can survive for several hours on objects like toilet seats or towels. But, for the most part, STD germs die soon after leaving the human body.

Because these germs generally survive only in mucous membranes, STDs are usually transmitted (spread) when an infected person's mucous membranes come in contact with another person's mucous membranes. This kind of membrane-to-membrane contact usually only happens during some form of sexual activity. However, it's not necessary for a male to ejaculate in order to pass the disease to his sex partner; any type of membrane-to-membrane contact can spread the disease. It is also possible to spread certain STDs from one part of the body to another with the fingers. For instance, touching a herpes sore and then touching your eye could lead to an eye infection (which could cause blindness). And touching an STD sore or discharge and then touching another person's mucous membranes could also spread the disease.

STDs can be also be transmitted in other nonsexual ways. For instance, certain STDs can be passed from an infected mother to her baby before or during birth. This can be very serious for the baby and may cause blindness, mental retardation, or other birth defects.

Candidiasis (yeast infections) is almost always spread in nonsexual ways. Improper wiping after a bowel movement may bring yeasts from a female's rectum into her vagina. In addition, yeasts normally live in some females' vaginas, though the natural acidity of the vagina keeps them in check. However, taking antibiotics, using birth control pills, being pregnant, or having diabetes may make the vagina less acid, allowing the yeasts to reproduce wildly and cause a vaginal discharge and other symptoms.

Although PID is usually the result of sexually transmitted germs moving up into the female pelvic organs, operations, abortions, and childbirth can also lead to PID. Trich, nonspecific vaginitis, nonspecific urethritis, and pubic lice can also be transmitted in nonsexual ways.

Though STDs can be spread in these nonsexual ways, most cases of STDs are the result of sexual activity. We should, however, mention that you can't get STDs from masturbating by yourself, from sitting clothed on someone else's lap, from a swimming pool or hot tub, or in any way other than the ones explained here or on the pages that follow.

The questions and answers in the following pages may help you understand more about STDs.

I heard that if you get a cold sore on your lip, it means you have herpes. Is this true?

In order to understand the answer to this question, you need to understand first that there are different types of herpes viruses and that they cause different kinds of diseases. Chicken pox, for instance, is caused by a herpes virus. The common cold sore, or fever blister, is also caused by another herpes virus, known as herpes simplex, type I (HSV-1), which results in blister-like sores in and around the mouth. Genital herpes is caused by a similar but different herpes virus, known as herpes virus, type II (HSV-2), which usually causes blister-like sores on or around the genital (sex) organs.

Having a cold sore only means that you "have herpes" in the sense that someone with chicken pox has herpes, that is, you have an infection caused by one of the herpes viruses. Having a cold sore *does not* mean you have the sexually transmitted disease known as genital herpes or just plain "herpes," as it is sometimes called.

Can you get an STD from kissing?

As a general rule, the answer to this question is no. However, there are some exceptions. Having oral-genital sex with someone who has a syphilis or herpes sore in his or her genital area could cause the sore to appear on your lip or mouth. Or, if you kissed a person who had one of these sores on the mouth or lip, you could get herpes or syphilis. (This is why it's not a good idea to kiss someone who has a sore on the lip, or to have oral-genital sex with a person who has a sore in the genital area.)

The only other exception is that it might be possible to get certain STDs from French-kissing (deep, open-mouth kissing where one or both people put their tongues in the other person's mouth). For instance, people can get gonorrhea germs in the back of the throat from oral-genital sex. So, if you French-kissed such a person, it would be possible to get the infection this way.

Can you get an STD from a toilet seat, a drinking glass, a towel, a wash cloth, or other object?

Except for STDs like pubic lice, which can live for a few days outside the human body, or trichs, which can survive for a number of hours, most STD germs die almost instantly when they leave the mucous membranes and are exposed to air. So, generally speaking, the answer to this question is no. In fact, in order to get an STD from a toilet seat, you'd have to put your mucous membranes in contact with the seat *immediately* after the seat had come in contact with the discharge or the mucous membranes of a person who had an STD. This, of course, isn't very likely to happen. It would be possible to get STD from an object like a drinking glass, towel, or wash cloth if it had *just* been used by a person with an STD sore, or an STD discharge. But, as a general rule, people don't get STDs from objects.

How can a person tell if he or she has an STD?
There are special medical tests to determine whether or not a person has an STD, and if so what kind. One way people find out that they have an STD is that they develop symptoms like the ones described above. The symptoms lead the person to see a doctor who tests him or her to see if the symptoms are being caused by an STD.

Because a person can have an STD without knowing it and because untreated STDs can lead to serious health problems, it is *vitally important* that anyone who's had contact with an infected person seek medical attention *right away*, regardless of whether or not they have symptoms. And people diagnosed as having an STD must inform *all* their sexual partners, so these people can be tested and, if necessary, treated. Even if the sexual partners don't have any symptoms, they must still be tested and treated.

What should you do if you think you might have an STD?
You should go straight to a doctor or clinic. Private doctors treat STDs and most Planned Parenthood clinics also provide free or low-cost STD testing and treatment. You can also get free testing and treatment from your county Health Department.

You don't need your parents' permission to be tested or treated, and no one will inform your parents that you have been. Doctors and the people who work at clinics are used to dealing with young people who have STDs. You don't need to feel embarrassed or ashamed to go for testing.

Even if you don't have symptoms, but think you may have had contact with an infected person, it's very important that you be tested. Even if your symptoms have disappeared, the germs could still be in your body causing damage, and you could still pass the infection to others.

Most STDs can be treated quite easily—usually with antibiotics—*provided they are treated right away*. But, if they go undetected and untreated, they can cause lasting damage to the body.

If you have questions regarding testing or treatment (or any other questions about STDs) you can call the National VD Hotline, 1-800-227-8922. This is a toll-free number, so there's no charge for the call and it won't appear on your phone bill. The call is confidential and you don't have to give your name, so don't hesitate to call.

Is there anything you can do to prevent getting an STD?
There are a number of things you can do to help prevent or at least cut down on your chances of getting an STD. First of all, personal hygiene is very important. You should wash your genitals every day and wear clean cotton underwear. Avoid deodorants, perfumes, and strong or scented soaps as they can irritate and dry out the genital skin, making it more susceptible to infection. Avoid synthetic underwear, tight jeans, and other tight clothing because they cut down on air flow and keep the genital area damp, making it more susceptible to infection. Females should always wipe from front to back, away from the vagina, when going to the bathroom, to avoid transferring germs from the rectum to the vagina.

Using condoms will help prevent STDs, though they do not offer 100% protection. Spermicides have also been shown to reduce the chances of developing STDs.

The cervical cap and the diaphragm also cut down the chances of a female developing certain types of STDs. But none of these methods offers 100% protection.

Above all, never have sex with a person who has STD symptoms—that is, unusual discharges, or rashes or sores on or around their sex organs. If you or your sexual partner currently has an STD, do not have any form of sexual contact again until the doctors says it's safe to do so.

Waiting until you're older before you start to have sex may also cut down on your chances of getting an STD. People who start their sex lives at an earlier age generally have a greater number of sexual partners in the course of their lives (and hence more STDs) than people who wait until they're older.

Choosing your sexual partners carefully is also important in preventing sexually transmitted diseases. If you don't know your sexual partner well, you don't know if that person is the type who'd inform you if he or she did develop symptoms later on. For this reason, it is always a good idea to use a condom when you start having sex with a new partner, when you are having sex with someone who has other sexual partners, or if you yourself have more than one partner.

STDs can lead to serious health problems, especially for women, so taking the preventive measures and precautions described above is very important.

AIDS

The letters in the word AIDS stand for Acquired Immune Deficiency Syndrome. It is a relatively new dis-

acquired (eh-CHOIR-ed)
immune (eh-MUNE)
deficiency (dee-FISH-n-see)
syndrome (SIN-drome)

ease. The first cases in this country were discovered in 1981. AIDS is considered an STD because it is most often spread through sexual intercourse. But because AIDS is different from other STDs and because it is such a serious disease, we decided to discuss AIDS in a special section of its own.

Scientists believes AIDS is caused by a virus. The AIDS virus attacks the immune system, the body's built-in defense against disease. The immune system keeps us healthy by destroying many of the disease-causing germs that get into our bodies and helps us to recover if we do become ill. The AIDS virus prevents the immune system from doing its job properly, so people with AIDS may become deathly ill from diseases that other people would recover from quite easily. People with AIDS may also develop certain rare, life-threatening illnesses that people with normal, undamaged immune systems would never have gotten in the first place. The AIDS virus can also infect the brain, causing serious and deadly brain diseases.

How Is AIDS Transmitted?

You may have heard all sorts of rumors about how AIDS is spread. If so, it's important to remember that the AIDS virus doesn't live *in* the air or *on* the things we touch, the way cold or flu viruses do. This means you can't get AIDS from what doctors call "casual contact"—that is, from coughs or sneezes, from eating food, from touching objects or people, or from being around an infected person. You can't get AIDS from normal everyday activities such as working at a job, attending school, using a public bathroom, taking a bath or shower, swimming in a pool, sitting in a hot tub, eating in a restaurant, shaking hands, using headphones, having someone whisper in your ear or breathe on you, hugging someone, or drinking from a glass or water fountain.

Scientists know that AIDS can't be spread through casual contact because, if it could be, there'd be many, many doctors, nurses, family members, and other people living with or caring for AIDs patients who would have come down with the disease. All of the people who've gotten the disease in this country have gotten it in one of the following ways:

1. *Sexual Intercourse:* Most cases of AIDS are spread through some type of sexual intercourse. Many people have the mistaken idea that infected females can't pass the disease to their male sexual partners, but this isn't true. People of either sex can pass the disease to their sex partners.

2. *IV Needles:* The second most common way in which AIDS is passed is through sharing needles used to inject illegal IV drugs such as heroin (smack), cocaine, "speed," or other "hard" drugs. When people use IV (intravenous) needles to "shoot up" (inject such drugs), some of their blood is drawn back up into the needle. Sometimes it's only a small amount of blood, too small to be seen. But, if a person uses a needle that has even a tiny amount of blood from an infected person, he or she can get AIDS.

   You can't, however, get AIDS from an injection given by a doctor, nurse, or health worker. These people use disposable needles or ones that have been properly sterilized, so there's no danger of getting AIDS.

   We should also mention the fact that there have been a very small number of cases in which a doctor, nurse, or other health care worker developed AIDS as a result of accidentally sticking themselves with a needle while drawing blood from or giving an injection of medicine to an AIDS patient.

3. *Blood Transfusions:* Although it is less common than #1 or #2 above, it is also possible for a person to get AIDS from having a transfusion of blood or blood products. Such transfusions are sometimes given before, during, or after an operation if a person has lost too much blood. People who have certain medical problems, such as hemophilia (a disease in which

hemophilia (HE-moe-FEEL-ee-ah)

the blood does not clot properly so that even a small cut or bruise can result in uncontrollable bleeding), may also be given transfusions. We now have a special test to make sure the blood or blood products used in transfusions are not infected with the AIDS virus. So nowadays, there is very little chance of a person becoming infected in this way. But those who had transfusions between 1976 and 1985 (when the test became available) could have gotten AIDS if infected blood or blood products were used in the transfusion. *A person can't, however, get AIDS from donating (giving) blood.*

We should also mention that there have been at least three cases where a nurse or other health care worker developed AIDS after accidentally spilling infected blood from an AIDS patient onto an open cut, sore, or break in the skin. This was, in effect, the same as a blood transfusion, for it allowed viruses from the infected blood to travel directly into the health care worker's bloodstream.

4. *Pregnant Woman to Infant:* An infected pregnant woman can pass the AIDS virus into her unborn baby's bloodstream because the mother and the developing baby share the same blood. It may also be possible to pass the virus during birth or through breast-milk. These are not, however, common ways of passing AIDS at the present time; less than 1% of AIDS cases in the United States as of 1987 were caused in this way.

What all this means is that if you haven't started having sex yet *and* you have never used illegal IV drugs *and* you have never had a blood transfusion, there's just no way you could have the disease. So, you can relax. But even if you are sexually active, there are things you can do to protect yourself from AIDS. Whatever you do, don't let fear keep you from learning the facts you need to know.

Exposure, Infection, and Disease

Young people often want to know if everyone who comes in contact with the AIDS virus actually gets AIDS. Just as people don't get colds or flu every time they come in contact with a cold or flu virus, neither does everyone who comes into contact with the AIDS virus get AIDS.

However, a lot of the confusion about AIDS stems from the fact that most people don't really understand the difference between coming in *contact* with a virus, becoming *infected* with the virus, and actually *developing* a viral disease. The table below gives some definitions we think are helpful in terms of understanding how any virus, including the AIDS virus, "works."

Phase 1: Exposure. Exposure means a person has come in actual physical contact with the virus. Exposure doesn't necessarily lead to infection, but it *may* lead to phase 2, infection.

Phase 2: Infection. Infection means the virus has actually moved inside some of the cells of the person's body. Any infected person is capable of infecting others. But being infected doesn't necessarily mean the person will develop symptoms. However, infection *may* lead to phase 3, disease.

Phase 3: Disease. Disease means the person has not only been exposed and infected, but has actually come down with symptoms. In such cases, we say the person "has" the disease.

We don't know how many of the people *exposed* to the virus will actually become infected. Nor do we know how many of those *infected* will actually come down with AIDS. At first experts thought that only about 20% to 30% of those infected would eventually develop symptoms. But recent studies suggest that this percentage may be much higher. Many experts are now afraid that a large number of those infected may eventually come down with AIDS or ARC, a related disease (see page 192).

Important Facts About AIDS
The following facts are important for anyone who hopes to understand AIDS:

- AIDS has spread at an alarming rate. In 1981, 321 cases of AIDS were reported in the U.S. By August of 1987, about 40,000 Americans had been diagnosed as having AIDS. By 1991, experts estimate that the total number of cases will have reached anywhere from 220,000 to 750,000 (or more).
- As of August of 1987, about 23,000 Americans had died of AIDS.
- The AIDS virus belongs to a certain category or type of rare virus. Scientists have never found a cure for any of the diseases caused by this class of virus, so they don't expect to find a cure for AIDS any time soon. (Some are afraid that a cure may never be found.) So far, no one has ever recovered from AIDS. Few who have been diagnosed as having AIDS have survived for more than five years.
- Some people infected by the AIDS virus develop symptoms within a few months; others don't develop symptoms for a number of years. It is not uncommon for the symptoms to take five years or even longer to show up.
- Experts estimate that as of 1987, one to two million Americans have been infected with the AIDS virus (though many of these people are not aware of this fact, since they haven't yet developed symptoms).

These facts explain why government leaders, doctors, health officials, as well as many other people, are so worried about AIDS.

The questions and answers on the following pages will help you understand more about AIDS. However, if you are a drug user, if you're already having sex, or if you're even thinking about it, you need more detailed information than we have room for in this book. I hope you'll read the book on AIDS that I wrote especially for young people like you. It's called *Lynda Madaras Talks to Teens About AIDS* (Newmarket Press, 1988). It's a short book, but it gives you all the information you need to protect yourself from AIDS. Reading it could literally save your life! You might also want to send away for some of the free pamphlets listed on pages

242–245 of this book, or look at some of the books and videos listed there.

The material in this section is based on the most up-to-date information that was available at the time this book went to press. But scientists are making new discoveries all the time. You can get the most recent, accurate information by calling the Public Health Service AIDS Hotline, toll-free, at 800-342-AIDS. There is no charge for the call. It won't appear on your phone bill and you don't need to give your name. A trained counselor will answer any questions you may have.

What kinds of symptoms does AIDS cause?
Some people don't have any symptoms at first, and they look and feel completely healthy. For others, the disease may begin with one or more of the following symptoms: swollen glands, extreme tiredness, loss of appetite; sudden and unplanned weight loss, night sweats, skin rashes, fevers, headaches, diarrhea, and white spots or a white coating on the tongue. Many of these symptoms can also be caused by more common diseases, including colds and flu. The difference is that AIDS symptoms tend to last much longer than you'd normally expect.

As the immune system breaks down, other diseases develop and cause other symptoms. For instance, many AIDS patients get a rare form of cancer that causes pink, brown, or purple lumps on the inside or outside of the body. Some get a rare pneumonia which causes coughing, chest pain, and difficulty in breathing. Some get brain diseases and have symptoms such as personality changes, loss of memory, and other signs of mental illness.

Some people with AIDS get sick and stay sick until they die. Others have periods of being quite healthy, followed by periods of sickness, then recovery, then sickness, and so on. Eventually, though, they are no longer able to recover.

What is ARC? How is ARC different from AIDS?
ARC stands for <u>A</u>IDS-<u>R</u>elated <u>C</u>omplex. Like people with AIDS, people with ARC have become infected with the AIDS virus and have developed symptoms. ARC symptoms tend to be less serious, though in some cases ARC patients may be quite ill and may even die. Experts estimate that 10% to 20% of the people with ARC will develop AIDS within five years.

Is there a test for AIDS?
Scientists hope to have a test that could detect the AIDS virus soon. Until then we only have the AIDS antibody test. *Antibodies* are substances that the immune system makes to try and destroy viruses or other disease-causing organisms. Different antibodies are made for each different type of germ. The AIDS antibody test involves taking a sample of the person's blood and studying it in a scientific laboratory to see if there are any AIDS antibodies. If there are, the test is positive. If there aren't, the test is negative.

But the AIDS antibody test only tells us whether the person has AIDS antibodies. It doesn't tell us whether the person will eventually develop symptoms. But people with positive antibody tests should not have babies or do anything else that might spread the disease to others.

If the antibody test is negative, doesn't this show that the person hasn't been infected with the virus?
Not necessarily. It usually takes four to eight weeks, and sometimes as long as six months, for a person to produce enough antibodies to show up on the test. So,

if a person became infected and had the test right away, before the antibodies had enough time to build up, that person might have a negative antibody test, even though he or she really was infected. Therefore, if you wanted to be certain you didn't have the virus, you would have to make sure you didn't do anything that could possibly expose you to the virus for six months before you had the test.

If it can take years to develop symptoms, how can scientists be sure that AIDS can't be passed through casual contact? Isn't it possible that people living with or caring for AIDS patients really have gotten the disease through casual contact, but that it just hasn't shown up yet?

These are good questions and ones that many people ask. Although it's true that it can take many years for the symptoms to show up, the antibodies show up fairly quickly.

Scientists have given repeated antibody tests over a period of many months, and even years, to thousands of family members, nurses, doctors, and others who have had casual contact with AIDS patients. Except for those who had used IV drugs, had blood transfusions, or had sex with an infected person, *none* of these people have had positive antibody tests. Therefore, scientists are sure the disease can't be spread through casual contact.

Could you get AIDS from a mosquito bite or from some other kind of insect bite?

No. For one thing, blood-sucking insects usually wait twenty-four hours or longer between feedings, and the AIDS virus would die long before this. Also, insects only withdraw blood. They don't inject blood into a person. Besides, if mosquitoes could spread the disease, we'd be seeing an unusually high number of AIDS cases in areas of the country where there are mosquitoes, and this isn't the case. There was a rumor about people in a town in Florida getting AIDS from mosquito bites, but it turned out not to be true. Scientists are quite certain that you can't get AIDS from insect bites.

I heard that infected people can have the virus in their saliva and tears, so couldn't the disease be passed through contact with these body fluids? If you were bitten by an infected person would you get AIDS? Can you get AIDS from kissing? How about French kissing?

We lumped these questions together because they have similar answers. It is true that the AIDS virus has been found in the saliva and tears of some AIDS patients.* However, this doesn't mean that AIDS can be transmitted by contact with tears or by a simple kiss. If people could get AIDS in these ways, there would be a lot more cases of AIDS among family members and health workers. Moreover, even when infected people do have the virus in their saliva, the actual number of viruses is very small. So, even if a person did get some saliva from kissing an infected person, there probably wouldn't be enough viruses absorbed through the mucous membranes of the mouth to cause the person to become infected.

Scientists are not entirely certain what would happen if a person who had an open sore or cut on the mouth kissed an infected person or if a person were bitten by an infected person. Open sores or cuts and bites that break the skin would allow any virus in infected saliva to travel directly into the person's bloodstream, so scientists can't rule out the possibility of the disease being

* Some kids in my classes have the mistaken idea that this means that the body is getting rid of the virus or that people could somehow spit or cry the viruses out of their bodies altogether. Neither of these things is true. Tears and saliva don't rid the body of the viruses. There will still be more viruses in the blood, constantly reproducing and making more viruses.

passed in these ways. However, we do know that there have been cases of people being bitten by AIDS patients, and that none of the people bitten have become infected. Nor do we know of anyone with an open mouth sore or cut getting AIDS from kissing. (Still, it's never a good idea to kiss someone while you have a sore or cut on your mouth—not just because of AIDS, but also because of other germs.)

There aren't any known cases of people getting AIDS from French kissing ("open mouth" kissing where one or both people put their tongues in each other's mouth). However, there are certain cells that can be found deep in the back of the throat that can carry the AIDS virus. So here again, scientists can't say that it's 100% impossible to get AIDS in this way.

Can people get AIDS from oral-genital sex?
Scientists can't be sure because the people who've gotten AIDS have usually had not just oral-genital sex, but other types of sex as well. Therefore, no one knows if oral-genital sex alone would transmit the disease. However, we know that the virus can live in vaginal secretions and in the semen of infected males, so most experts feel it may be possible that oral-genital sex can transmit the disease.

Is it true that in this country the majority of persons with AIDS are male homosexuals or bisexuals, and male and female heterosexuals who use illegal IV drugs? Does this mean heterosexuals who don't use drugs and haven't had blood transfusions don't really need to worry about AIDS?
In order to understand the answer to these questions, you need to know that a male *homosexual* is a person who has sex with other males; a male *bisexual* is a person

homosexual (hoe-moe-SEC-shoe-ul)
bisexual (bye-SEC-shoe-ul)

who has sex with other males and also with females; a *heterosexual* is a person who has sex with people of the opposite sex. (All of this is explained in more detail in the next chapter, so you might want to jump ahead before you read the answer to these questions.)

The answer to the first question above is yes. The majority of cases of AIDS reported in this country have occurred among male homosexuals and bisexuals, or among male or female heterosexuals who use IV drugs.

However, the answer to the second question is no. Despite what some people think, AIDS is not a "homosexual" or "drug-users" disease. In fact, in other parts of the world, such as Africa, AIDS is more common among heterosexuals than among homosexuals, and it is equally common among males and females. Even though the majority of cases in this country so far have occurred among homosexuals, bisexuals and drug users, this *does not* mean the disease will continue to be confined to these groups. In the future, experts expect to see larger numbers of heterosexuals who've never had transfusions and who don't use IV drugs getting AIDS. Indeed, many such people may already have been infected with the virus, but because it can take so long for symptoms to develop, we haven't yet seen large numbers of such people coming down with AIDS. Just about anyone who is sexually active needs to be concerned about AIDS and to take steps to protect against the virus.

What do people mean when they say, "Nowadays, when you have sex with someone, you're not only having sex with that person, but with everyone he or she has had sex with and those people's sex partners, too?"

They mean that even though your sex partner isn't a

heterosexual (HET-er-oh-SEC-shoe-ul)

male homosexual or bisexual, isn't a drug user, and isn't someone who's ever had a blood transfusion, he or she may have had sex with someone who is, or that person's previous sex partners may have had sex with such a person. In either case, your sex partner may have gotten the virus, and even though he or she may not have symptoms, he or she could pass the virus on to you.

How can I protect myself from getting AIDS?
When young people ask us this question, the first thing we tell them is: DON'T USE ILLEGAL IV DRUGS! Don't use them even once. In fact, stay away from all illegal drugs, because using these drugs increases the chances that a person will get "hooked" on drugs and will eventually go on to use IV drugs. (Those who do use IV drugs should *never* share needles.) Don't have sex with anyone who uses these drugs or with someone who has sex with drug users.

The second thing we tell young people who ask this question is that AIDS is mainly a sexually transmitted disease. Therefore, abstinence, that is, waiting until you're older or until you're married before you have sex, is, of course, the most effective way of preventing AIDS. We also remind young people not to make the mistake of thinking that having sexual intercourse is the only way to have a deep, meaningful, pleasurable, and romantic sexual experience with someone else. Hugging, touching, kissing, and other activities that don't involve the exchange of body fluids are "safe" ways of expressing and sharing sexual feelings.

Finally, if you're going to have sex, USE CONDOMS. Some young people have a hard time believing that this advice applies to them. They don't think that anyone they'd be having sex with could possibly have the virus, so they don't see why they need to use condoms. But nowadays just about anyone could have the virus. Unless your sex partner answers "no" to the following questions and you're *sure* he or she is telling the truth, you *must* use condoms:

1. Have you ever had a transfusion of blood or blood products?
2. Have you ever used illegal IV drugs?
3. Have you ever before had any type of sexual intercourse (including oral-genital sex)?
4. Will you be using IV drugs or having intercourse with anyone else during the course of your sexual relationship?

It's important to remember that just as condoms may not be 100% effective in preventing pregnancy, they also may not be 100% efective in preventing AIDS. For example, condoms that are too old or are stored improperly may break or leak. Moreover, people don't always use them properly. If you're not absolutely certain that you know how to buy, use, and store condoms, you should contact your local Planned Parenthood or the AIDS hotline (800-342-AIDS). If you don't know the facts about condoms or if you feel too shy or embarrassed to talk to a potential sex partner about condoms, we suggest you read our book, *Lynda Madaras Talks to Teens About AIDS* (Newmarket Press, 1988). In fact, we urge all young people who are sexually active or are even thinking about having sex to read this book. It could literally save your life!

OTHER HEALTH PROBLEMS:
URINARY INFECTIONS, JOCK ITCH,
ACHING BALLS, HERNIA, ETC.

In addition to asking about STDs, the boys in my classes also ask questions about other health problems. Here are some of the questions they ask:

I've never had sex, but I have symptoms like you said you get from STDs. I have pain; it burns when I urinate; and sometimes, a little bit of stuff leaks out of my penis. If it's not an STD, what is it?

There are a number of diseases other than STDs that can cause these kinds of symptoms. For example, urethritis, an infection of the urethra, or urinary tract, can cause these symptoms. Sometimes urethritis germs are passed through sexual contact, but you can also pick up these germs in other ways.

What is jock itch?

"Jock itch" or "jock rot" is a fungus infection caused by wearing clothes that are too tight or that don't let the air circulate freely. It causes redness, soreness, and itching on the genitals and the inside of the thighs. Rubbing cornstarch on the area may be enough to cure the problem, but sometimes special medication from the doctor is needed to clear it up. Keeping the area clean and dry, washing your clothes frequently, and avoiding tight clothing will help prevent the problem.

What would happen if a boy only had one testicle?

Most males are born with two testicles. Every once in a great while, someone is born with only one. Or, a man or boy could have some sort of injury or accident that could crush one testicle so badly that it had to be surgically removed.

If, for one reason or another, a man has only one testicle, the other testicle takes over for the missing one and produces enough sperm so that he'll still be able to make a woman pregnant. His sex life and everything else about him will be completely normal.

What is an undescended testicle?

Before a boy is born, his testicles are up inside his body. Once he is born, they descend (come down) into his scrotal sac. Sometimes one or both testicles don't descend, and the boy has what doctors call an *undescended testicle*. (At times, cold weather, a cold bath, excitement, or extreme physical activity will cause one or both of a boy's testicles to retract, that is, to draw up close to his body for a while. But this is a temporary condition. It's not the same as an undescended testicle.)

No one knows what causes an undescended testicle, but luckily, doctors do know how to cure it. Sometimes the doctor can use medicine to make the testicle descend; at other times it's necessary for the boy to have an operation.

I was masturbating and I didn't want to get semen all over my pajamas, so I put my finger over the top of my penis just as I was ejaculating so nothing would come out. And nothing did, but for the last couple of days I've had this pain in my penis and this milky stuff has come out. What should I do?

This kind of problem is not at all unusual among boys. It's called *retrograde ejaculation*, and it happens when the semen is prevented from spurting out through the opening in the glans of the penis during ejaculation. In older men, there are certain medical problems that cause retrograde ejaculation. But in boys, it usually happens when the boy is masturbating, and for some reason or another doesn't want to ejaculate. So, he puts his hand or thumb or something over the opening in the penis as he's about to ejaculate, as the boy who asked this question did.

Retrograde means "going backward." In retrograde ejaculation, the semen can't come out the end of the penis, so it travels backward down the urethra. It may be forced up the tube that leads to the bladder, which can cause the urine to be cloudy for some time afterwards. The semen may also be forced into the prostate

retrograde (RET-row-grade)

gland. In either case, there may be pain and discharge from the penis.

In some instances, the symptoms will clear up all by themselves, but often a doctor's care is needed. Although it may be embarrassing for a boy to tell the doctor that he's been masturbating and to explain how the retrograde ejaculation happened, it's important to see the doctor if you have pain, a milky discharge, or milky urine. If the semen is forced up into the prostate gland, the tissues of the gland could become irritated and susceptible to infection. The doctor can treat such infections with antibiotics and, if necessary, with pain-killers. For these reasons, it is not a good idea to prevent your ejaculate from coming out the end of your penis.

My penis is sort of swollen and red and my foreskin is stuck, so I can't pull it down. What's wrong?
Sometimes these symptoms are caused by a foreskin that's too tight or a foreskin that has become stuck to the glans of the penis. This can be quite uncomfortable and may cause pain and swelling. Such problems can be cured by circumcision, and there are sometimes other ways of treating the problem. It's important, though, that you see a doctor and have the problem taken care of.

I have pain in my genitals, but I don't really want to see a doctor. I've never had sex, so it can't be an STD. What could it be?
It's a bit difficult to say what could be causing this problem without knowing more. We've already explained about urethritis, retrograde ejaculation, and foreskin problems—any of which could cause pain in the genitals. In addition, here are some other possibilities:

- *Swollen glands:* There are glands in the genital area called lymph glands. It's possible, even if you've never had sex, to get an

lymph (limf)

infection in these glands, which can result in pain and swelling. Treatment with antibiotics usually cures the problem.

- *"Aching balls":* This isn't really a disease or a medical problem, but it can cause pain in the testicles or genital area. Aching balls happens when a boy has an erection for a long time without ejaculating or without having his penis get soft again (because he's still sexually stimulated). For example, a boy could have a long kissing session with his girlfriend that could cause him to have a prolonged erection that might result in aching balls. Even after his erection goes away, the achy feeling may persist. It happens because the blood has been trapped in the erect penis for such a long time. Although it may be uncomfortable for a while, it's not a serious problem and doesn't require a doctor's treatment. The achy feeling goes away in, at most, a few hours.

- *Hernia:* A hernia occurs when part of the intestines bulge through a weak spot in the wall of the abdomen. If it happens in the lower part of the abdomen, it can cause pain in the genital area. If untreated, hernias can cause serious medical problems. They are usually treated by surgery in which the doctor repairs the weak spot.

- *Twisted testicles:* No one knows just why this happens. It is rare, but when it does occur it is a medical emergency. It usually follows some physical exertion and causes extreme pain, nausea, vomiting, and fever. It requires immediate surgery.

I have these funny pimples (white) on my penis. I've never had sex. Why does this happen?

It's most unlikely that you'd get an STD unless you have some sort of sexual contact with another person. But the skin of your penis, just like the skin on other parts of your body, is subject to all sorts of pimples, bumps, warts, irritations, birthmarks, scars, and so forth. The white, pimple-like bumps may just be blocked oil glands in the skin of the penis. Such pimples aren't anything to worry about. Of course, anytime you have some problem that bothers you, it's always a good idea to have it checked out by your doctor.

hernia (HER-knee-ah)

I have this lump in my scrotum. It doesn't hurt; what is it? Can boys get cancer of the scrotum?

Most lumps or bumps in the scrotum are the result of cysts, which are collections of fluid. Some of these cysts will go away by themselves; others require an operation. Although the vast majority of lumps in boys' scrotums are not serious, it's a good idea to get them checked by a doctor.

It is possible for boys to get cancer of the testicles and scrotum, but it is very rare. When it does happen, the first symptom is often a lump in the scrotum. This doesn't meant that *all* lumps (or even most lumps) in the scrotal sac are cancerous lumps. But because a few are, it's important to have any lump checked out by a doctor. Although it can happen to older and younger men, testicle cancer is most often found in young men between the ages of twenty and thirty-five. The earlier it is found, the easier it is to cure. For this reason, doctors recommend that boys and men practice a regular testicular self-exam (TSE), which is explained in Illustration 34.

SEXUAL CRIMES

When we talk about sexual intercourse in class, I often find questions about sexual crimes in the "Everything You Ever Wanted to Know" question box. So, we want to discuss this topic, in case you too have questions about these things.

Parents sometimes worry about bringing up the topic of sexual crimes with their children because they don't want to scare them. Many parents want to protect their children from even hearing about such terrible things. This is understandable, but the fact of the matter is,

cysts (SISTS)

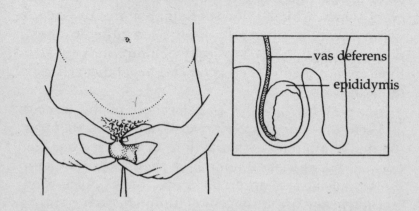

Illustration 34. Testicular self-exam. It's best to examine your scrotum right after a hot bath or shower. The scrotal skin is most relaxed at this time, and the testicles can be felt more easily. Examine each gently with the fingers of both hands. Put your index and middle fingers on the under side of the testicle and your thumb on the top. Roll your testicle gently between your thumb and fingers, feeling for a small lump about the size of a pea. Repeat this procedure for the other testicle.

You should learn what the epididymis feels like at the back of the testicle so that you won't confuse it with an abnormality. If you do find anything abnormal, most often it will be a firm area on the front or side of the testicle.

Testicular cancer constitutes fewer than 1 percent of all cancers, but it is one of the most common cancers in men aged twenty to thirty-five years. It's forty times more likely to occur among men in whom the testes never descend to the scrotum or descend after the age of six.

Most testicular cancers are first discovered by men themselves. Since testicular cancers found early and treated promptly have an excellent chance for cure, learning how to examine your testes properly can help save your life. It really doesn't take much effort to search for those small lumps, and you only have to do it once a month. Use the simple testicular self-examination (TSE) procedure shown here.

sexual crimes do happen. We feel that the best way to protect children from sexual crimes is to make sure they know about these things and are prepared to handle the situation if they become victims of a sexual crime.

The three types of sexual crimes we'll be talking about here are rape, incest, and child molesting.

Rape

Rape means forcing someone to have sex against his or her will. It can happen to anyone—to young children, to adults, to people of any age. Most rape victims are females, and most rapists are males. Theoretically, it's possible for a woman to hold a gun to a man's head and force him to have intercourse with her, or for a woman to force a person (male or female) to have oral-genital sex with her, or something like this. It is also possible for a male to be raped by another male. By and large, though, rape cases involve a male raping a female.

If you are a victim of rape, the most important thing is to get help right away. Some rape victims are so upset by what's happened that they just want to go home and try to forget the whole thing. But a rape victim needs medical attention as soon as possible. Even if the victim doesn't seem to have any serious injuries, there could be internal injuries that need medical attention. The victim also needs to be tested to make sure that he or she hasn't gotten a sexually transmitted disease from the rape. If the victim is a woman, she needs a test to make sure she isn't pregnant and she may want to take the morning-after pill to prevent pregnancy. (These tests are one reason why a victim shouldn't bathe or shower before seeking medical attention). And, a rape victim should seek help because he or she will need support to recover emotionally as well as physically.

If you are a rape victim, there are a number of ways to go about getting help. You can go to a hospital emergency room or call the police, who will take you to the hospital. There are Rape Hotlines in most big towns and cities. You can find the number of the hotline closest to your home in your telephone directory or by calling the information operator.

Incest and Child Molesting

Incest involves one member of a family being sexual with another family member. It may include anything from touching, feeling, or kissing the sex organs to actual sexual intercourse. Of course, it isn't incest when a husband and wife do these things with each other. But when it happens between other family members, it's called incest.

Most victims of incest are girls who are victimized by their fathers, stepfathers, brothers, or some other male relative, although it is also possible for a girl to be victimized by a female relative. Boys can also be victims of incest. When incest happens to a boy, it may be either a female or a male relative who victimizes him. Incest can happen to very young children, even to babies, as well as to older children and teenagers.

Brothers and sisters often engage in some form of sex play as they're growing up, which may involve "playing doctor" or pretending to be "mommy and daddy." This kind of sex play between brothers and sisters is very common. It isn't always considered incest and it isn't necessarily a harmful thing. But being forced or pressured to have sexual contact with a brother or sister *is* incest, and it can be very harmful.

Incest isn't always a forced thing, like rape. Because of the older person's position in the family, he (or she) may be able to pressure the child into doing sexual things without actually having to use force. Most incest victims are so bewildered by what's going on that they simply don't know how to stop it or prevent it from happening again.

Child molesting, like incest, may involve anything from touching, feeling, or kissing the sex organs to actual sexual intercourse. (The word *molest* means to bother or to harm). But child molesting is different from incest because the person doing the molesting isn't a family member. It may be a complete stranger, a friend of the child's parents, or some other older person. Boys as well as girls may be victims of a child molester.

If you are a victim of incest or child molesting, the most important thing to do is to *tell someone*. This can be a difficult thing to do, particularly if you are an incest victim.

The logical people to tell are your parents. (Of course, in cases of incest by a parent, you need to tell the other parent). However, some parents have trouble believing their children at first. If, for whatever reason, your parents won't believe you, you might tell another relative—an aunt or uncle, a grandparent, an older sister or brother—whom you feel *will* believe you. Or you could tell another adult—a teacher or counselor at school, a friend's mother or father, your minister or priest, or any other adult you trust. You can also call the Child Abuse Hotline. The number is 800-422-4453. This number is toll-free, which means you don't have to pay for the call and it won't show up on your phone bill.

The people who answer the phones there are specially trained and they understand what you're going through. (Some of them have been victims of sexual crimes themselves.) You don't have to give your name, and what you say is entirely confidential, so don't hesitate to call.

Victims of incest or child molesting often find it hard to come forward and tell someone. Sometimes the person who committed the crime has made the victim promise to keep it a secret. But, there are some promises and some secrets a person needn't keep, and this is definitely one of them. Or, the victims may find it hard to tell someone because they think that what happened is somehow their fault, or that they're to blame because they didn't stop it from happening. But, this just isn't true. These crimes are *always* the fault of the older person. The victim is *never* to blame and is *never* at fault in any way. Some victims don't tell because they are afraid the person will harm them or get back at them for telling. But, the police or other authorities can make sure the victim is *fully protected*.

Incest victims sometimes hesitate to tell because incest is a crime, and it's possible that telling could get the person who has committed the crime into trouble with the police. Even though most victims hate what's been done to them, some of them still don't want to see a relative sent to jail. Although involving the police may seem like a horrifying idea, it will be better for everyone in the end and will protect any brothers or sisters who may also be suffering abuse. Besides, those who commit incest aren't always sent to jail. If possible the judge sends the person for some form of psychiatric treatment, while at the same time making sure that you are protected from further abuse.

Some incest victims don't tell because they're afraid that the family will break up, their parents will get divorced, or things will get worse than they are. But, if incest is going on, things are already about as bad as they could be. The victim and the other family members also need help in dealing with the situation. However, no one can get the help they need unless the victim has the courage to take the first step and tell someone.

Most victims of incest and child molesting feel a mixture of anger, embarrassment, and shame. This can also make it hard to come forward and tell someone. But you have a right to protect yourself from being touched in ways that don't feel right to you. So even though you may feel embarrassed, it's important to tell someone.

On a Lighter Note

When we went back and reread this chapter and the previous one, we were a little worried about how it sounded. All this talk about things like miscarriages, stillbirths, birth defects, AIDS and other sexually transmitted diseases, and sex crimes isn't exactly upbeat or cheery. Even though we think it's important to give our readers the kind of information that's in these chapters, we thought to ourselves, "Gee, kids who read this might feel like a ton of bricks just fell on their heads."

In other words, we were afraid that these chapters might make kids feel worried, upset, or depressed. Reading about so many negative things, one right after the other, can be a bit hard to take. We want to remind you that most women don't have miscarriages or stillbirths; most have completely trouble-free pregnancies and give birth to beautiful, healthy babies. And most people never have to face problems like rape, incest, child molesting, or AIDS. Although people can and do get sexually transmitted diseases, in most cases, they can be easily cured, especially when they're treated properly. So you shouldn't let the negative things in these chapters make you terribly worried. They're only a small part of the story.

CHAPTER 9

Romantic and Sexual Feelings

If a girl is thirteen and she's had her period and all she ever thinks about is boys and sex, is this normal?

I think I might be sex-crazy or something. I mean, I'm always thinking about girls, fantasizing, and I masturbate a lot, like almost every day. Do you think I'm okay?

These questions came out of the "Everything You Ever Wanted to Know" question box. Questions like these often come up because, as we go through puberty, many of us experience stronger romantic and/or sexual feelings than ever before in our lives. For some of us this means spending time imagining a passionate romance with a special someone, or having sexual fantasies. For some it means having the urge to masturbate more often. For some it means getting interested in the opposite sex, having crushes, or having a boyfriend or girlfriend.

These romantic or sexual feelings can be very strong. At times, it may even seem as if romance and sex are all you can think about! Some young people get so wrapped up that it's a bit scary for them. If, like the boy and girl who asked the above questions, you've been worried about your strong romantic or sexual feelings, it helps to know that these feelings are perfectly normal and natural and that a lot of people your age are going through the same thing.

Besides questions like ones above, there are also questions like these:

> How come all the other girls think about boys and getting dates and stuff and I don't even want to go out or have boyfriends or anything?

> My friends are always talking about girls and sex and everything. But, I'm just not interested in girls in a romantic way yet. Do you think there's something wrong with me?

When boys and girls ask questions like these, I explain that although puberty is a time of strong sexual or romantic feelings for many young people, not everyone experiences these feelings. Some boys and girls are more involved in sports, school, music, a job, or some other aspect of their lives. Just as we each have our own personal timetable of development when it comes to the body changes of puberty, so we each have our own personal timetable when it comes to romance and sexual interests. If you've worried that there's something wrong with you because everyone else your age is madly in love or all wrapped up in the opposite sex and you aren't interested in such things, you can stop worrying. There's nothing wrong with you. Your personal timetable is just different from theirs.

The boys and girls in my classes are curious about

anything and everything having to do with sex, and they're especially curious about the kinds of romantic and sexual feelings that young people have when they're growing up. We've talked about fantasies and masturbation elsewhere in this book, and we'll mention these topics again in this chapter, particularly in the last section which deals with the difference between feeling private and feeling guilty about sexual matters.

But having fantasies and masturbating are basically private things that you do by yourself. In this chapter, we'll be talking more about your sexual and romantic feelings that involve other people. We'll be talking about romantic and sexual relationships and about things like crushes, dating, falling in love, kissing, necking, petting, and other topics that come up in our classes. Of course, there isn't room in this one chapter to fully cover these topics, but we hope we can answer at least some of your questions. Before we get started talking about romantic and sexual feelings and relationships, though, we'd like to say a couple of things about friendships.

"JUST FRIENDS"

You may be one of those kids who becomes interested in the opposite sex in a new way, develops crushes, begins having boyfriends or girlfriends, or even starts dating during your puberty years. Or you may not experience these things. Either way, you'll undoubtedly notice that boy-girl relationships start to change as puberty rolls around and that things are quite a bit different than when you were younger.

When we're small children no one makes much of a fuss over the fact that two kids of the opposite sex are friends. Occasionally, people will make cracks about "puppy love," but it's just not a big deal if a little boy and girl play together, are best friends, spend the night at each others' houses, and so forth. As puberty approaches, though, things change. Suddenly, it's no longer okay to spend the night at your best friend's house if your best friend happens to be someone of the opposite sex. The other kids at school or the adults around suddenly start assuming that you must be more than "just friends," that you "like" each other in a romantic, boyfriend/girlfriend sort of way.

At least, the kids in my classes often complain that it's harder to be "just friends" after you reach a certain age. Here's what one girl in my class had to say about this:

> I'm going to Paul's Halloween party on Saturday, and my brother keeps teasing me, "Oh, you like Paul, you're in love with Paul." Well, I do like Paul, but not like that. All of a sudden, you can't just be friends with a boy. It's got to be boyfriend or girlfriend, like you're all romantic with each other.

An eleven-year-old boy who'd been friends with a girl since they were little kids had this to say:

> I went over to Hilary's house to spend the night, and we were swimming in the pool. These girls who live next door came over and they were saying things like, "Oh, you're playing with a girl. Oh, you're staying overnight at a girl's house. Oh, that's weird. You must be gay."
>
> Donny, age 11

Many kids complain about this sort of teasing and about people automatically assuming that a friend of the opposite sex is more than "just a friend." So, in class, we talk about how to handle this problem. Here's some advice we've come up with together:

- Just ignore the teasing and rumors.
- Explain to people that you *are* "just friends."
- Talk to your friend about it so the teasing or rumors don't make you feel uncomfortable around each other or affect your friendship.
- Don't worry about it too much because, when you're older, opposite-sex friendships aren't such a big deal anymore.
- "Turn things around" and act like the people who are teasing you are the ones who are weird for not being able to be friends with someone of the opposite sex.
- Take a "so what" attitude. After all, who cares if they think you're madly in love with your friend?
- Tell them why you think it's fun or a good idea or whatever to be "just friends" and what you get out of being close friends with someone of the opposite sex.
- Realize they may be jealous because they'd really like to have an opposite-sex friendship.

We think that the above suggestions are pretty good ones. So, if you're having problems in this way, take some of this advice, and don't let "the romance thing" keep you from enjoying an opposite-sex friendship.

CRUSHES

Of course, sometimes we are interested in romance. In fact, many boys and girls develop crushes. Having a crush means having romantic or sexual feelings towards a certain, special someone. Crushes can be very exciting. Just thinking about or catching a glimpse of the person you have a crush on can brighten your whole day, and you may spend delightful hours imagining a romance with him or her.

Sometimes boys and girls develop crushes on someone who isn't very likely to return their affections—a film star, a rock singer, a teacher or other adult, or a friend of an older brother or sister. These sorts of crushes can be a safe and healthy way of experimenting with romantic and sexual attractions—no matter how much we may pretend otherwise, deep down we know that this person is unattainable. So, we don't have to worry about real-life problems like what to say or how to act. We're free to imagine what we like, without worrying about whether that person will be attracted to us. In a way, having a crush on someone unattainable is a way of rehearsing for the time in our lives when we will have a real-life romance.

But having a crush on someone unattainable can also cause a lot of suffering. One year some of the girls in my class developed crushes on a certain rock star. They plastered their bedroom walls with posters, wore buttons with his face printed on them, pored over fan magazines, and generally had a great time sharing their feelings about him with one another. When the rock star got married, they were, naturally, somewhat disappointed, but one girl was more than disappointed. She was really upset. She had gotten too involved in her crush, and the rock star's marriage was devastating for her. If you find yourself developing a serious crush on someone unattainable, it helps to remind yourself from time to time that your crush isn't very realistic and that this person isn't very likely to return your affections.

Not all crushes are unrealistic. You may develop a crush on someone near your own age whom you actually know through school, church, temple, or some other group. If that person shows an interest in you as well, the crush can be especially exciting. But yearning after a person who doesn't return your affections can be painful. If you find that your crushes are causing you problems, it helps to find someone—a friend, a parent, a teacher, another adult, or a counselor—with whom you can discuss your feelings.

When we talk about crushes and being romantically or sexually interested in a certain, special someone you've actually met or know, I'm often asked questions like these:

How do you find out if someone likes you? How do you let someone know you like them?

There are basically two ways: You can do it on your own, or you can have a friend do it for you.

If you decide to have a friend do it, you'll want to pick someone you really trust, or next thing you know it will be all over school! It's often easier to let someone else do the talking for you. But keep in mind that, if you do this, you don't have very much control over what's being said. Suppose, for example, you only want your friend to bring up your name in a roundabout way and see how this other person reacts. Instead, your friend might tell this other person that you're madly in love with him or her!

For these reasons, many people prefer doing it on their own. You can let someone know you like him or her by being friendly, starting conversations, going out of your way to be around that person, asking the person to go out with you, or simply telling the person how you feel. You can also find out if a person likes you by watching to see if that person does any of these sorts of things to *you*.

Regardless of whether you tell the person yourself or have a friend do it for you, make sure it's done in private and not in front of your other friends or classmates. Otherwise, the person may be so embarrassed that he or she may say they don't like you even if they really do!

DATING

As young people move through puberty and into their teen years, many begin dating. This can be fun and exciting, but it can also create problems. For instance, you may want to date before your parents think you're old enough. Or you may not feel ready to date, and your parents or friends may be pushing you into it. You may have trouble deciding whether you want to go steady with one person or go out with lots of different people. If you've been dating one person regularly and decide you want to date others, you may have problems in ending your steady dating relationship. Or, if your steady boyfriend or girlfriend decides to change the relationship, you may have a hard time coping with this. On the other hand, if you want to date and no one is interested in going out with you, you may feel rather depressed.

Here again, if you're having problems that relate to dating, it might be helpful for you to talk them over with someone you respect and trust. One of your parents, another adult you trust, a friend, or an older brother or sister might be someone you could talk to. You might also want to take a look at our book, *Lynda Madaras' Growing Up Guide for Girls* (Newmarket Press, 1986), which talks about these issues. Even though this book was written for girls, lots of boys have found it useful, too. In addition, it might be helpful for you to hear some of the questions that come up in my classes about this topic.

Suppose that you'd like to date, but you never have and you're beginning to wonder if you ever will?
If the other kids you know have already started dating, but you haven't, you may get to feeling that these things won't ever happen to you. If so, it helps to

remember that, just as we each have our own special timetable of development when it comes to the physical changes of puberty, so we each have our own time-tables when it comes to romantic matters. It can be awfully hard if your personal timetable is moving along more slowly than other people's. But the fact that you're getting a slow start doesn't mean that you won't ever start dating. It may take a while, but eventually, you'll start dating too. We guarantee it!

Remember, you've got many years ahead of you. It doesn't really matter if you start dating when you're only twelve years old or not until you're twenty. What's important in the long run is that you feel good about yourself.

What if every time you ask someone out, the answer is "no"?
If you've asked a girl out a number of times and she keeps saying "no," then you may just have to face the fact that she doesn't want to go out with you. It can be difficult to know exactly how many times you should ask before giving up altogether. Partly, it will depend on what she says when turning you down. If she tells you that she's already dating someone else or simply isn't interested in you, then that's a pretty clear sign that you should stop asking. But, if she says, "I'm sorry, but I'm busy," or doesn't give a clear reason for saying "no," you might want to try again. Perhaps she really is busy, but would like to go out with you another time. But if you've tried a few times and have gotten this kind of reply, you might want to say something like, "Is there a time when we could get together?" The answer to this question will usually give you a clear idea of whether it's worth your while to keep asking this person out.

If you've asked a number of different girls out and

all of them have said "no," you may begin feeling awfully discouraged. You may even start to feel that there's something so wrong or so horrible about you that no one will ever say "yes." But, before you allow yourself to feel down and discouraged, think for a moment about who you're asking out—maybe they're the wrong people! Are you only asking the best-looking or most popular girls? If so, this may be part of your problem. For one thing, the best-looking and most popular girls may already have lots of people asking them out, so your chances aren't as good as if you asked someone less popular or not-totally-gorgeous. Besides, the fact that someone is popular or pretty doesn't necessarily mean you're going to have a great time with her. What's more important is whether she's nice, whether the two of you could be comfortable with each other, whether you could have fun together. The person's inner qualities are a lot more important than other qualities like being popular or good-looking.

You might also ask yourself how well you know the person you're asking out. If you're asking someone you hardly know, this may be a big part of the reason you keep getting turned down. If you take the time to get to know someone and to let her get to know you first, you'll have a better chance of having her say "yes" when you ask for a date.

It might also be helpful for you to have a mutual friend check things out before you ask for a date. Your friend can give you an idea of how she might respond. If she isn't interested, you'll save yourself the discouragement of being turned down again. In addition, you might ask some of your friends who they think you should ask for a date. People love to play matchmaker, and your friends may come up with someone you wouldn't have thought of on your own. They may even know someone who's been dying to go out with you! So don't hesitate to enlist your friends' help.

Suppose you want to date, but your parents say "no"?
Young people usually choose to handle this problem in one of three ways: 1) Sneak around behind their parents' backs; 2) Go along with their parents' rules and wait until their parents say they're old enough; 3) Try and change their parents' minds. Let's look at each of these choices.

Sneaking around just isn't a good idea. If you get caught, you may get into a lot of trouble, and your parents may find it hard to trust you in the future. Even if you don't get caught, you'll probably feel awfully guilty about lying, which isn't much fun. So in the end sneaking around really isn't worth the price you may have to pay.

On the other hand, it can be awfully hard to go along with your parents' rules and wait until you're older, especially if there's a special someone you'd like to date. But parents usually aren't trying to be mean or unfair. They're trying to protect you from "getting in over your head" by dating at too young an age. Maybe they're right. If your parents say "no," ask yourself these questions: Are the other kids my age allowed to go out? Would I really lose anything by waiting until I'm older?

If your honest answer to these two questions is "no," then perhaps waiting is the best choice for you. If, however, you feel that your parents are being too strict or too old-fashioned, you might want to consider the third choice, changing their minds.

This may not be easy, but it's worth a try. For starters, find out exactly why they've made these rules. What are they worried about? Once you hear them out, you may be able to come up with a compromise. If, for instance, your parents think you're too young to go out on a solo date, maybe they'd allow you to go on group dates. Or, if they won't allow dates for the movies, perhaps they'll allow you to go to a boy–girl party or invite someone to your house.

How do you know if it's really love?
Once they begin dating, many young people fall in love, or at least what they think might be love, so they ask questions like the one above.

Emotions can't be weighed or measured and different people have different ideas of what it means to be in love. So, we can't give you a definite answer to this question. But we can share with you some of our thoughts on the subject.

We think it's important to recognize the differences between infatuation and true love. *Infatuation* is an intense, exciting (and sometimes confusing or scary) fireworks kind of feeling. You may be so wrapped up in your infatuation that it's hard to think about anything else. People sometimes mistake infatuation for love. But infatuation usually doesn't last very long; true love does. You may start out being infatuated and have it grow into true love. Or, the infatuation may pass and you may discover that you weren't really "right" for each other, after all. In addition, you don't have to know someone very well in order to be infatuated. But in order to truly love someone, you have to know that person (both their good qualities and bad ones) very well. In addition, infatuation can happen all of a sudden. True love takes more time.

Regardless of whether your relationship starts with the fireworks, infatuation-kind-of-feeling or develops more slowly and gradually, sooner or later love relationships go through a questioning stage, where one or both of you begin to question whether this relationship is really a good one. During this questioning stage, one or the other of you may decide to end the relationship. In our opinion, it's only after you go through this questioning stage and decide to stay together that you're really on the road to true love.

HOMOSEXUAL FEELINGS

This is another topic that always comes up when we talk in class about the sexual and romantic feelings people have during their growing-up years. *Homo* means "same." Having *homosexual feelings* means having romantic or sexual thoughts, fantasies, dreams, attractions, or crushes that involve someone who is the same sex as we are. Many boys and girls have homosexual thoughts or feelings, or actual sexual experiences with someone of the same sex, while they're growing up.

If you've had homosexual feelings or experiences, you may realize that this is quite normal, and you may not be at all worried about it. Or, you may feel somewhat confused or upset, or even downright scared, about having these kinds of feelings or experiences. Perhaps you've heard people making jokes or using insulting slang terms when talking about homosexuality. If so, this may have caused you to wonder if your homosexual feelings or experiences are really okay. Perhaps you have heard someone say that homosexuality is morally wrong, sinful, abnormal, or a sign of mental sickness. If so, this, too, may have made you wonder or worry about your own feelings. If you've heard any of these things (or even if you haven't), we think it will be helpful for you to know the basic facts about homosexuality.

Although almost everyone has homosexual feelings

or experiences at some time or another in their lives, we usually consider people to be homosexuals only if, as adults, their strongest romantic and sexual attractions are towards someone of the same sex, or most of their actual sexual experiences involve someone of the same sex.

Both males and females may be homosexuals. Female homosexuals are also called *lesbians*. "Gay" is a non-insulting slang term for both male and female homosexuals. There have been homosexuals throughout history—some very famous. People from any social class, ethnic background, religious affiliation, or economic level may be homosexual. Doctors, nurses, lawyers, bus drivers, police officers, artists, business people, ministers, rabbis, priests, teachers, politicians, football players, married people, single people, parents: you name it—all sorts of people are homosexuals.

The majority of adults in our society are *heterosexual* people (hetero means "opposite") whose strong romantic and sexual attractions are towards the opposite sex and whose actual sexual experiences mostly involve the opposite sex. However, about one in every ten adults is a homosexual. Although an adult is usually considered either a homosexual or a heterosexual, this doesn't mean that he or she doesn't sometimes have feelings or experiences in the other direction. Very few people are *strictly* homosexual or *strictly* heterosexual.

Now that you know a bit about homosexuality, you might want to read some questions that the students in my classes have asked and the answers to these questions.

Is homosexuality morally wrong? Is it unnatural, abnormal, or a sign of a mental sickness?

In the past, many people felt that homosexuality was

lesbians (LES-be-anz)

sinful or abnormal, and there are still some people who think it's morally wrong or a sign of mental illness that needs to be cured by a psychiatrist. However, nowadays, many people no longer believe this. They feel that it's a personal matter, that some people just happen to be homosexuals, and that being homosexual is a perfectly healthy, normal, and acceptable way to be.

What's a bisexual?
A bisexual is a person who is equally attracted to males and females and whose sexual activities may involve either sex.

If a person has a lot of homosexual feelings or fools around with someone of the same sex while growing up, will this person be a homosexual as an adult?
Having homosexual feelings and experiences while you're growing up has *nothing at all* to do with whether or not you'll be homosexual as an adult. Some of the young people who have homosexual feelings and experiences while they're growing up turn out to be homosexuals as adults and some turn out to be heterosexuals. Some adult homosexuals had homosexual feelings while they were growing up; others had heterosexual feelings; still others didn't have strong feelings one way or the other as they were growing up.

Can a person know for sure that they're gay even though they're still young?
Yes. At least, some gay adults say that they knew they were homosexuals when they were teens, or even when they were very small children.

How can I find out more about homosexuality?
If you would like more information about homosexuality, you might be interested in some of the books

listed at the back of this book on pages 242-245. You can also contact the Gay and Lesbian Community Service Center, 1213 North Highland Avenue, Los Angeles, CA 90038. They publish a newsletter called REACH, which is written for and by gay teens, and they will send you a free copy in a plain envelope if you request it. In addition, their Temenos Youth Outreach program sponsors a pen pal program, and on Fridays and Saturdays from 7:00 p.m. to midnight, West Coast time, they have a talk line for gay teens (213-462-8130).

Is there anything else I should know about homosexuality?
Yes. You should know that male homosexuals and male bisexuals are at higher risk of getting AIDS, a deadly sexually transmitted disease that is passed through contact with infected body fluids such as blood, semen, urine, or feces. Homosexual activity that involves the exchange of these body fluids could lead to AIDS if one or the other person has the AIDS virus in his or her body. So, males who have sexual contact with homosexuals or bisexuals should pay special attention to the section on AIDS on pages 185-198 of this book. The Gay and Lesbian Health Center listed also has a free pamphlet and information on "safe sex."

MAKING DECISIONS ABOUT HOW TO HANDLE YOUR ROMANTIC AND SEXUAL FEELINGS

Once young people begin going out, they often find themselves faced with questions about how to handle the strong romantic and sexual feelings they may be having. When two people are attracted to each other, they quite naturally want to be physically close. Being physically close may mean something as simple as holding hands or kissing goodnight after a date. Or, it may mean more than this. Physical closeness may even include something as intimate as sexual intercourse.

Some young people don't have much trouble in deciding what kind of physical closeness is right for them or in making decisions about "how far" they want to go in terms of physical intimacy. Such young people have strong moral or religious beliefs or other values that guide them in making these sorts of decisions. But other young people aren't sure what's right or wrong when it comes to deciding how far to go. And even those who *are* sure sometimes have a difficult time sticking to their beliefs once they're actually in a romantic situation. So, I usually spend a good deal of time, especially in my classes for older boys and girls, discussing the topic of making decisions about how to handle romantic and sexual feelings. There isn't enough space here to cover everything we discuss in class, but in the following pages we'll answer some of the most frequently asked questions.

If there were one set of answers that everyone agreed with, it would be easy to answer these sorts of questions, and our job as sex education teacher/writers would be much easier. But, it's not that simple: Different people have different ideas on these issues, and many of them feel quite strongly about their point of view. So we try to present these many different opinions as thoroughly as possible, and explain why people feel the way they do, without "taking sides" one way or the other. We think it's important for young people to hear all sides of a question and come up with their own answers, rather than just going along with someone else's opinion. For example, some young people answer questions about how to handle their sexual and romantic feelings based on what they think "everyone else" is doing. Not only are they often wrong about "everyone else" is doing, but the fact of the matter is that *just because "everyone else" does it, does not mean it's right for you.*

Or, to take another example, some young people don't think through these issues on their own and just "go along" with what their parents or their religions say is right or wrong. Now, please don't misunderstand what we're saying here. We're not saying that you shouldn't follow your parents' or your religion's teachings or rules. In fact, we think parents and religions have excellent advice that's well worth following. But we've found that young people who just accept what they've been taught without thinking things through for themselves frequently run into problems when they're actually in situations where they have to make decisions about "how far" to go. Oftentimes, they aren't able to stick to the rules they've been taught. The rules sort of "fall apart" or "cave in" in the face of the tremendous pressure to experiment sexually that's often put on young people. We think this happens because the rules weren't really "theirs" in the first place; they come from someone else. Not until you consider all the different viewpoints and decide for yourself what rules to follow will the rules become truly your own. And it's not until the rules are truly your own that they become rules you can live by.

I'd like to have a girlfriend, but is someone my age (eleven) old enough to have sex? I'm twelve and there's a certain girl in my class that I like, and she likes me, too. I'm scared of having sex, though. What should I do? We kissed goodnight after our first date. I want to go out with her again, but what if I get her pregnant?

It's usually younger boys and girls who ask these sorts of questions. When I first heard questions like these, I was a bit shocked that boys and girls who were so young seemed to be asking questions about whether they were ready for sex. However, in talking further with the young kids who asked these sorts of questions, I realized that the reason they were asking these questions was often because they had very mistaken ideas about physical intimacy. Some of them thought that kissing or being physically close in other ways happens almost as soon as you get involved with someone, or at least very quickly—perhaps even before you've had a chance to get to know each other. Some thought that going on a date means you have to, at the very least, kiss the person goodnight or perhaps even go further. Some even thought that having a boyfriend or girlfriend automatically means that you're going to have sexual intercourse with that person.

These things just aren't true, but it's easy to see how kids get these mistaken ideas. In the books we read, it often seems as if two people who meet on one page will be madly kissing each other on the next page. In the movies, it sometimes seems as if two perfect strangers take one look at each other, and the next thing we know they're in bed together!

But in real life, things don't usually happen quite like this. A romantic relationship usually goes through several steps or stages of physical closeness before sexual intercourse occurs, if indeed the relationship ever goes that far.

So please don't be confused by what you read in books or see on TV or in the movies. Dating or having girlfriends doesn't mean that you have to have sex or kiss or even just hold hands. Above all, remember that when it comes to romance and sex, you're in charge and you don't have to do anything that doesn't feel right for you.

What is French-kissing? What's the right way to French-kiss?

French-kissing, which some people call tongue-kissing, means that one or both people put their tongues in the other person's mouth while kissing. Some people like French-kissing; other don't and choose not to do it. There is no "right" or "wrong" way to French-kiss. Some people just put the tip of their tongue into the other person's mouth. Others put more of their tongue in; still others manage to get their tongues in each other's mouth at the same time. There just aren't any specific rules about this.

What is necking? What is petting?

Necking—or "making out" as some people call it— means having prolonged kissing sessions. Different people define "petting" differently. Some people use the phrase "petting above the waist" or "light petting" to describe a situation in which a male feels or fondles a female's breasts. "Petting below the waist" or "heavy petting" means touching or rubbing the other person's genital organs. Some people further divide petting into "petting outside or over your clothes" and "petting inside or under your clothes."

What is mutual masturbation? What do people mean when they say "doing everything but"? What does "going all the way" mean?

Mutual masturbation means masturbating while another person also masturbates, or masturbating each other. "Doing everything but" means that although two people stop short of actually having sexual intercourse, they engage in other forms of physical closeness such as heavy petting; getting naked or partially naked and hugging, rubbing, or touching each other's bodies; mutual masturbation; oral-genital sex; or other intimate sexual contact. "Going all the way" means having sexual intercourse, that is, the male putting his penis in the female's vagina.

Is it all right to kiss on your first date? Is it wrong to get into necking? How about petting? How far is "too far" to go? Where should you draw the line? Is it okay to "do everything but," as long as you don't "go all the way" and have sex?

As we explained earlier, if everyone agreed upon these issues, these would be easy questions to answer. But, of course, they don't. For instance, some people think it's not right to kiss on a first date, while others think it's perfectly okay to do so. Some people think necking is okay; others don't. Some people think it's "sinful" to go beyond necking or, perhaps, light petting. Some don't think this is morally wrong, but are afraid that young people might get "too carried away" or "too turned on" and wind up going further than they really meant to. Other people have still other opinions on these issues, and some people just aren't certain exactly *how* to answer these sorts of questions.

Young people's answers to the sorts of questions listed above are strongly influenced by their personal situations—by their parents' values, their friend's opinions, their religion's teachings, their own moral beliefs, and their own emotional feelings. These influences affect each of us differently, but we think there are some basic guidelines that are helpful to anyone facing these questions, regardless of their personal situation, morals, or values:

1. Whether it's French-kissing, petting, or going further, don't let yourself be rushed into anything. Do only what you're really sure you want to do. After all, you have many years ahead of you; you can afford to wait until you are sure.
2. Ask yourself how you feel about this other person. Is this someone you trust? Will this person start rumors or gossip about you? Are you doing these things because you really

care about this person or simply because you're curious to try these things? Young people are naturally curious about how it feels to neck, pet, or do some of these other things, but remember that it may not be as pleasurable if you're only doing it out of curiosity.

3. Ask yourself *why* you want to do this. Your real reasons may not have much to do with your feelings about the other person or even with your curiosity about these things. You may actually be hoping to prove you're grown up, trying to become more popular, or afraid you'll "lose" him or her if you don't. But agreeing to kiss, neck, pet, or go further for these reasons doesn't solve any of these problems. In fact, it may create new ones.

4. Don't pressure someone into doing something he or she doesn't want to do. This pressure may take the form of a boy persuading a girl to go further than she really wants to, or of a girl acting like a boy isn't "manly" if he doesn't want to kiss or doesn't try to get her to go further.

5. Don't allow yourself to fall for a "line," such as: "If you liked me, you'd neck with me"; "If you truly cared about me, you wouldn't say no"; "If you don't, I'll find someone else who will"; "Everybody else is doing it." If someone hands you one of these lines, turn the line back on them: "If you truly cared about me, you wouldn't pressure me"; "Prove you love me by not pushing me"; "So go ahead and find someone else"; "If everybody else is doing it, you shouldn't have much trouble finding someone to do it with you."

6. Don't assume you know what the other person is thinking—*ask*. Many boys and girls get involved in necking, petting, or other sexual activities even though they don't really want to, just because they think the other person wants or expects to do these things. But this isn't always the case. Sometimes neither of you really wants to, so talk things over first.

7. Don't be afraid to say "no." Sometimes young people get involved in doing something because they're afraid they'll hurt someone's feeings if they refuse. We're all taught not to be selfish or hurt another's feelings. But your sexuality is one aspect of your life you have a right to be selfish about, so if you don't want to, it's okay to say "no."

8. Don't be too hard on yourself if you make a mistake and afterwards find that you've done something you wished you

hadn't. Learning to make decisions about how to handle your romantic and sexual feelings is just like learning anything else: you're bound to make mistakes. Remember, too, that if you have done something you regret, you can always decide to behave differently in the future.

How old should you be before you start having sex? Should you wait until you're married? Is it okay to have sex if you're really in love, even though you're not married? Are teenagers mature enough to handle sex? Why do people make such a big fuss about sex? I mean, if two people want to have sex, why shouldn't they just go ahead and do it?

Even though each of these questions is phrased a bit differently, they are all about the same thing—when is it all right for a person to have sex and when isn't it? Once again, there isn't just one set of agreed-upon rules, and different people have different ideas on this subject.

Some people feel it's acceptable for two people to have sex with each other as long as they're both adults or have reached a certain age. Some of these people consider a person to be an adult once he or she has reached a specific age, such as eighteen or twenty-one. Others think you're an adult once you're out on your own, that is, once you're no longer living with your parents and/or you're earning your own living and supporting yourself. Still others have what we call the "legal" point of view. They feel it's all right for people to have sex as long as they're over the legal age limit, which varies from state to state.

However, for most people, it's not *how old* you are that's the important thing. For instance, many people feel that you shouldn't have sex until you're married, regardless of your age. People who have the "wait until you're married" point of view may have this opinion for a variety of different reasons. For some, it's religious. They feel that the Bible tells us very clearly that people should not have sex unless they're married to each other. Others are concerned about what will happen if an unmarried couple has sex and a pregnancy results. Such people are often morally opposed to abortion. They feel that a decision to have sex isn't just a decision between two people but a choice that involves the responsibility for a third person, the baby that might be conceived. For this reason, they feel that you shouldn't have sex until you're married and are able to take on the responsibility of raising a child.

There are also other reasons why people have a "wait until you're married" point of view. One man we interviewed, whom we'll call Charlie, explained his reasons particularly well. Charlie was not a religious person, but as he explains, he decided not to have sex until he was married:

My wife and I waited until we were married to have sex, which is unusual nowadays. But I think it was a good decision. Maybe if we'd had sex with other people or with each other before we were married, we'd have been more experienced or knowledgeable. But learning about sex together made it that much more special. We didn't have to worry if either of us was as good as the other lovers either of us might have had before.

By being willing to wait until we were married, I felt I was showing my wife that it wasn't just sex that I wanted from her but real, true love and a lifelong commitment. And she was showing me the same thing. We really trusted each other, and that made us feel safe enough to really let go. We didn't have to worry that if we did it wrong or it wasn't great the first time that it would be all over. And, in fact, it wasn't so great the first time. It was kind of awkward and embarrassing. But I knew and she knew that we'd both be around tomorrow. This trust and commitment made us able to grow to be better lovers than we might otherwise have been.

While some people feel strongly about waiting until you're married or until you've reached a certain age, others put more emphasis on maturity or on the nature of the relationship. For instance, some people feel it's all right to have sex if you're really in love. Some say it's all right even if you're not in love, as long you're really committed to a serious, long-term relationship. Some say it's all right as long as you're both mature enough to handle it.

Of course, it's not always easy to know for sure if it's really love, just how serious or long-lasting the relationship will be, or whether you're really mature enough to handle it. But people who have these kinds of guidelines are concerned about the emotional feelings involved in sex. Having sexual intercourse involves very intense emotional feelings, and it's very easy for people to be hurt. When parents don't want teenagers to have sex, many times they're concerned not only about morality or the possibility of pregnancy, but also about the emotional pain that can result when the relationship ends. Also, as Charlie pointed out, sex is something that takes some time to work out. If two people aren't in love or in a long-term relationship that guarantees that the other person will be around to work things out with, one or both people may suffer emotionally.

One young woman we interviewed had something especially interesting to say about why she thought it was important to wait to have sex until you were involved in a serious relationship:

> I have girlfriends who think if you get into heavy petting and all that with a boy, it's stupid or artificial or something not to go all the way and have sex with him. They say sex isn't such a big deal. Maybe I'm too romantic or too idealistic, but

> I think sex *is* a big deal, or should be. I want it to be very
> deep and very emotional. . . . I know you can go around
> having sex all the time and it *won't* be a big deal for you. If
> you do that too much, though, I think you get, well, hard
> and cold and kind of callous. It's like you deaden yourself:
> you're no longer even capable of having it be deep or emo-
> tional.

There are also some people who don't place much
importance on being in love or in a serious relationship.
These people feel that if two people are attracted to
each other and want to have sex, then it's perfectly
acceptable for them to do so. Such people often feel
that society is "too uptight" or "too hung up" about
sex. They argue that sex is normal and natural and that
people should be free to enjoy it whenever they want
to, provided, of course, that both people consent to do
so. Some people even go so far as to say that it's all
right for two people to have sex even if they've just
met or hardly know each other. However, not everyone
who approves of casual sex is quite this casual about
it.

As we've explained, there are many moral, religious,
and emotional reasons why people don't feel that casual
sex is a wise idea. There are also health reasons. Having
casual sex increases your chances of getting sexually
transmitted diseases (STDs). STDs can have serious,
and in the case of AIDS, even deadly, consequences.
Because of these health issues, many people today feel
that casual sex is just far too risky.

So far, we've talked about people who have one certain viewpoint or another, but there are also many people who simply aren't sure how they feel about the
question of when it's all right for people to have sex.
If you're one of these, you might find it useful to talk
this over with other people. In the end, only you can

answer these questions and make your own decisions about how to handle your sexuality.

Don't (as many young people do) automatically rule out your parents as people to talk to. You may be surprised to find that your parents struggled with these same questions when they were your age. Young people often don't talk about sexual decision-making with their parents because they already know that their parents' attitudes are more conservative or stricter than theirs. But even if this is so, your parents may have good reasons for feeling the way they do. And even if you don't totally agree with them, they might have things to say that could prove useful to you. You might also talk with other people, an aunt or uncle, a sister or brother, or an older friend.

SEXUALITY: FEELING PRIVATE/FEELING GUILTY

Even though we haven't actually used the word *sexuality*, we've been talking about sexuality throughout this chapter—and in fact, throughout this whole book. Some people think the word sexuality only applies to sexual intercourse, but it also includes such things as your general attitudes about sex, feelings about your changing body, romantic and sexual fantasies, masturbation, childhood sex play, homosexual feelings, crushes, hugging, kissing, petting, and being physically close in other ways.

Feeling Private

Most people feel private, shy, or even a bit embarrassed about some aspect of their sexuality. Some young people, for instance, become very modest during puberty, and no longer feel okay about family members seeing

sexuality (SEK-shoo-AL-eh-tee)

them nude. Some feel embarrassed asking questions or talking about the changes happening in their bodies. Some feel very private about starting their periods or having wet dreams and don't want their families or friends to know that these things have happened.

Private feelings can also center around romantic and sexual feelings or activities. Some kids are shy about the fact that they have a crush. Others feel embarrassed about their fantasies or about homosexual feelings. For most, masturbation is something that's very private. Young people may also feel shy about things like kissing, necking, petting, and other kinds of physical closeness. Some feel embarrassed even talking about these things, let alone actually doing them.

Some kids even worry about the fact that sexuality is such a private thing for them. But, feeling private, shy, or even a bit embarrassed about sexuality is completely natural. It doesn't mean that you're "hung up" or "uptight" or that there's something wrong with you. It just means that you're normal!

Feeling Guilty

There is, however, a difference between feeling *private* about your sexuality and feeling *guilty* about it. Some kids don't just feel private, shy, or embarrassed, they also feel guilty, ashamed, "dirty," or otherwise bad about some aspect of their sexuality.

When young people tell us they're having these guilty feelings, we suggest that they ask themselves if what they're feeling guilty about is something that is (or could be) harmful to themselves or others. If it's not, then our advice is to try and let go of the guilty feelings. If, on the other hand, it is something that's harmful, our advice is to make amends (if possible), to stop doing whatever it is that has caused the guilty feelings, and to decide not to do it in the future.

Even when a person *has* done something harmful, it's often something that's not too serious. For instance, you might feel guilty if you'd been flirting with your best friend's steady. But this isn't really all that serious. At least, it's not as serious as the kind of situation described by a fifteen-year-old boy who was feeling guilty about having pressured his girlfriend to go further than she really wanted to:

> Necking is as far as she'd ever go because of her moral standards. I kept pushing and got her to, well . . . not actual intercourse, but further than she wanted to go. I didn't force her or anything. I was coming on strong, though. Now I feel like some kind of pervert, and I can tell she doesn't feel good about herself. It's changed things between us. We're not so close.

This boy had done something that was harmful to his girlfriend's good feelings about herself and to his own good feelings about himself. It also hurt their relationship.

In other cases, the harm may be even more serious. If, for example, you didn't tell a sex partner that you had a sexually transmitted disease, or if an unwanted pregnancy resulted from the fact that you didn't use contraception, then the harm done could be quite serious indeed. Generally speaking, the more serious the harm, the harder it is to deal with the guilt. And, even though you've changed your behavior and done what you can to make amends, this doesn't mean your guilt will go away completely.

It's important to remember that human beings are, after all, *human*. We do make mistakes. If you've done what you can to make amends and change your behavior, then it's important to forgive yourself and get on with your life.

We also want to remind you of the fact that different people have different ideas about what is or isn't harmful. Take, for example, masturbation, which is something many young people feel guilty about. Personally we think masturbating is a perfectly normal, perfectly healthy thing to do. Unless it goes against a person's moral principles (in which case it could be a harmful thing for that particular person), we usually advise young people who are feeling guilty about masturbating to try and relax and let go of the guilt. However, some people see things quite differently. They believe that masturbation is sinful or morally wrong and that people do themselves harm in a moral sense by masturbating. Because of these beliefs their advice would probably be just the opposite of ours. They might advise young people to stop masturbating, and to decide not to masturbate again in the future.

How people react to situations where they feel guilty will depend, then, not only on how serious any harm done may be, but also on their ideas as to what is or isn't harmful. It's also possible for young people to feel guilty about doing something that few people, if any, would consider harmful at all. For instance, one sixteen-year-old girl who wrote to us said:

> If I just kiss a boy goodnight I feel so ashamed, not while I'm kissing but afterwards. I know it's not normal to feel so guilty, yet I do. How can I get over feeling so guilty?

This girl felt guilty and ashamed simply for kissing a boy good-night. And, judging from the letters we get, she's not alone. Some kids feel guilty even though they haven't actually *done* anything at all. For example, some boys and girls have told us that they felt not just shy or embarrassed, but also ashamed, of the fact that they've gotten their periods or had wet dreams.

Kids who feel this ashamed—or, for that matter, any young people who are feeling guilty about their sexuality even though they haven't done anything harmful—may find it helpful to think about *why* they feel this way. Often it's because some important person (often a parent) or group (maybe a religion, a government, or just society in general) has taught or influenced them to feel this way. Until fairly recently in our history, most people in our society had *very* negative attitudes about sexuality. In your great grandparents' day, sexual thoughts and feelings were often considered evil, the work of the devil. Sexual desires were considered impure or unclean, especially in women. Women who felt sexual urges or who enjoyed sex were considered abnormal, sick, or perverted. Many people felt it was sinful even for married people to have sex, unless they were trying to have a child.

Of course, times change and so do people's attitudes. Today, most people in our society have more positive attitudes about sexuality, but there are still many people who have very negative, or at least somewhat negative, attitudes about sexuality. Parents who have these attitudes may pass them on to their children. Even though parents may not actually come out and say "sexuality is bad," they may pass these attitudes on in other ways. A parent might, for instance, get upset when a little baby touches his or her sex organs and move the baby's hand away or even slap them. This may give the baby the idea that sex organs are "nasty" or "dirty" and that it's "wrong" or "bad" to touch them. Thus, when that baby grows up, he or she may feel ashamed about menstruation or wet dreams or may feel guilty about masturbating.

When you think about it this way, it's really not surprising that some kids feel guilty about sexuality even though they haven't actually done anything that is harmful to themselves or others. It can be very difficult for these young people to let go of their guilty feelings. But, being aware of where these feelings come from can help. People can and do learn to work past their guilt. So, if you're feeling guilty even though you haven't done anything harmful, perhaps you should think about why you're feeling this way so that you, too, can learn to enjoy your sexuality.

A Few Final Words

You're growing up, and growing up isn't always an easy thing to do, but it's important to remember that growing up has its more positive sides. We are becoming sexual beings as we move through puberty and into adulthood. Sexuality is a rich and meaningful part of our lives, a source of deep joy and contentment, and puberty, despite the problems it may present, is an exciting time in our lives. It is a time of many "firsts"—first period, first date, first kiss, first love, first job, first driver's license. It is a time when we begin to become our very own independent selves. We hope that this book has helped you to understand more about your puberty and to enjoy it all the more.

FOR FURTHER READING

BOOKS FOR YOUNG CHILDREN

Ideally sex education should begin at a very early age. One way to introduce the topic is through some of the excellent picture books for young children. The following are among our favorites and are appropriate for four- to eight-year-olds.

Sheffield, Margaret and Bewley, Sheila. *Where Do Babies Come From?* (New York: Knopf, 1973).
  This book explains puberty, sex, conception, pregnancy, and birth in terms that even a very young child can understand. It is sensitively done and beautifully illustrated.

Waxman, Stephanie. *What Is a Girl? What Is a Boy?* (New York: HarperCollins, 1989).
  This frank and forthright book, illustrated with nude photos of infants, children, and adults, deals with the physical differences between the two sexes.

BOOKS FOR OLDER READERS

Alyson, Sasha and Fletcher, Lynne Y. *Young, Gay & Proud* (Boston: Alyson Publications, 1991).

A young person's guide to what it means to be gay; considered by many to be the best answer book for young gay people.

Bell, Ruth. *Changing Bodies, Changing Lives: A Book for Teens on Sex and Relationships* (New York: Random House, 1988).

A fine book, representing many points of view through quotes from teenagers themselves. The section on teenage pregnancy is especially good, and the one on mental health, depression, and suicide is outstanding. The book is geared toward the fifteen- to nineteen-year-old age group, but it could be valuable for younger and older people as well.

Calderone, Mary S., M.D. and Johnson, Eric W. *The Family Book About Sexuality*, rev. ed. (New York: HarperCollins, 1990).

Designed for the whole family, this book talks about how sexuality begins when we are only tiny babies, and how it develops through puberty and adulthood, and even into old age.

Comfort, Alex and Jane. *The Facts of Love: Living, Loving, and Growing* (New York: Ballantine, 1986).

This book covers many of the same topics dealt with in *Changing Bodies, Changing Lives*, but it is aimed at younger adolescents. More conservative parents may be more comfortable with this book than with the much franker presentation in *Changing Bodies*.

The Diagram Group. *Woman's Body: An Owner's Manual* and *Man's Body: An Owner's Manual* (New York: Bantam Books, 1978, 1983).

Excellent books that have chapters on the sex organs and sexuality. They also cover other parts of the body, illness, body care, fitness, nutrition, and a lot more.

Gardner-Loulan, Joann; Lopez, Bonnie; and Quackenbush, Maria. *Period* (San Francisco: Volcano Press, 1981).

This excellent picture book deals with menstruation and is especially useful for introducing preteens to the topic. The illustrations feature all ethnic groups and even handicapped kids (which most books don't).

Madaras, Lynda and Area. *My Body, My Self: The "What's Happening to My Body?" Workbook for Girls* (New York: Newmarket Press, 1993).

The companion volume to *The "What's Happening to My Body?" Book for Girls*, this workbook/diary is filled with factual information, quizzes, and checklists, offering adolescent girls ages 9 to 15 an ideal opportunity to explore and set down in writing their feelings about the changes they are going through. Includes quizzes, checklists, exercises, illustrations.

Madaras, Lynda and Area. *My Feelings, My Self: Lynda Madaras' Growing-Up Guide for Girls* (New York: Newmarket Press, 1993).

For pre-teens and teens, a workbook/journal to help girls explore their changing relationships with parents and friends; complete with quizzes, exercises, letters, and space to record personal experiences. Includes drawings and bibliography.

Madaras, Lynda and Saavedra, Dane. *The What's Happening to My Body? Book for Boys* (New York: Newmarket Press, 1984).

This is a book that a teenage friend and I wrote for boys about puberty. Needless to say, we think it's a pretty good one. Although it was written for boys, many girls and parents have read it and told us they learned a lot from it.

Planned Parenthood. *Kids Need to Know*.

Kids Need to Know is an information kit for parents and teens that includes booklets and pamphlets on topics such as sexuality and birth control. The kit is available from the Information and Education Department, Planned Parenthood, 1316 Third Street Promenade, Suite B5, Santa Monica, California 90401.

INFORMATION ABOUT AIDS

Madaras, Lynda. *Lynda Madaras Talks to Teens about AIDS* (New York: Newmarket Press, 1988).

Designed for teens aged fifteen through nineteen, many of whom may already be sexually active. Includes straightforward information on methods of transmission, high risk groups, and prevention through safe sex practices.

The National Public Health Service has a toll-free AIDS Hotline, 1-800-342-AIDS. In addition, there are some free pamphlets you can obtain by sending a self-addressed, stamped envelope to: AIDS and Children, Department of Health Education, New York University, 715 Broadway, New York, New York, 10003.

INDEX

(Page references in italics refer to illustrations.)

Lynda Madaras' growing-up books are highly recommended by reviewers, doctors, educators, librarians, and readers for their conversational tone ("Conversational, matter-of-fact, honest"—*Washington Post*) and coverage ("Madaras tackles some of the hardest subjects with the aim of provoking discussions rather than conveying her own point of view"—*Kirkus Reviews*).

THE "WHAT'S HAPPENING TO MY BODY?" BOOK FOR GIRLS: *A Growing Up Guide for Parents and Daughters.* Lynda Madaras with Area Madaras. Foreword by Cynthia W. Cooke, M.D.—304 pages; 44 drawings; index.

THE "WHAT'S HAPPENING TO MY BODY?" BOOK FOR BOYS: *A Growing Up Guide for Parents and Sons.* Lynda Madaras with Dane Saavedra. Foreword by Ralph I. Lopez, M.D.—288 pages; 34 drawings; index.

Over 500,000 copies have been sold of these two best-selling puberty education books for 8- to 15-year-olds, their parents, and other concerned adults. They include information appropriate for this age level about AIDS, other sexually transmitted diseases (STDs), and birth control. The Girls book covers the body's changing size and shape, menstruation, breasts, changes in reproductive organs, and includes a chapter on puberty in boys. The Boys book includes chapters on changing size and shape, hair, perspiration, pimples, voice changes, the reproductive organs, sexuality, puberty in girls, and much more.

MY BODY, MY SELF FOR GIRLS: *The "What's Happening to My Body?" Workbook.* Lynda Madaras and Area Madaras—128 pages; 7¼" x 9"; paperback.

With over 100 quizzes, checklists, and journal entries, this workbook companion encourages girls to address head on their questions and concerns about their changing bodies. Everything affected by the onset of puberty is covered.

MY BODY, MY SELF FOR BOYS: *The "What's Happening to My Body?" Workbook.* Lynda Madaras and Area Madaras—112 pages; 7¼" x 9"; paperback.

Packed with drawings, cartoons, games, checklists, quizzes, and innovative exercises, this book encourages boys to address head on their concerns with their body, body image, height, weight, growth, hair, voice changes, reproductive organs, sexuality, emotional problems of puberty, diet, and health.

MY FEELINGS, MY SELF: *Lynda Madaras' Growing-Up Guide for Girls.* Lynda Madaras with Area Madaras—160 pages; resource guide; 7¼" x 9"; paperback.

Focuses on relationships, feelings, self-knowledge, and problem-solving with parents, handling peer pressure, and making friends. Filled with quizzes, exercises, letters, and information to help girls explore what it feels like to be growing up.

LYNDA MADARAS BOOKS FOR PRE-TEENS AND TEENS
(AND THEIR FAMILIES, FRIENDS, AND TEACHERS)

Order from your local bookstore, or write or call:
Order Department, W. W. Norton, Inc., 500 Fifth Avenue, New York,
NY 10110; (800) 233-4830; Fax (800) 458-6515

Please send me the following books by Lynda Madaras:

THE "WHAT'S HAPPENING TO MY BODY?" BOOK FOR GIRLS
_____copies at $11.95 each (trade paperback)
_____copies at $18.95 each (hardcover)

THE "WHAT'S HAPPENING TO MY BODY?" BOOK FOR BOYS
_____copies at $11.95 each (trade paperback)
_____copies at $18.95 each (hardcover)

MY BODY, MY SELF FOR GIRLS
_____copies at $11.95 each (trade paperback)

MY BODY, MY SELF FOR BOYS
_____copies at $11.95 each (trade paperback)

MY FEELINGS, MY SELF (Lynda Madaras' Growing-Up Guide for Girls)
_____copies at $11.95 each (trade paperback)

For postage and handling, add $3.00 for the first book, plus $1.00 for
each additional book. (New York State residents please add 8.25% sales
tax.) Please allow 4 to 6 weeks for delivery.

I enclose a check or money order, payable to Newmarket Press, in the
amount of $_____.

Name_____

Address_____

City / State / Zip_____

Special discounts are available for orders of five or more copies. For
information contact Newmarket Press, Special Sales Dept., 18 East 48th St.,
New York, NY 10017; (212) 832-3575 or (800) 726-0600;
Fax: (212) 832-3629.